PRAISE FOR THE BURNED-OUT HEALER

The Burned-Out Healer – A Path to Trauma Release and Reconnection to Self is a very important book. It addresses the challenge of energy workers and spiritual healers— of burnout, of giving too much—and offers step by step solutions. This book is not just for energy workers and spiritual healers—this is a book for those involved in any healing and health care profession.

Ines Simpson
Creator of The Simpson Protocol Hypnosis

Jacquie creates the roadmap for healers to help themselves and become congruent with healing others. A must buy for anyone in the healing arts.

Tim Horn, PhD
Certified Hypnotist and Instructor

This book will be like salve to a wound for healers who over-extend themselves. It clearly shows how the solution lies within us, as does the problem and how taking accountability for our energy reserves will return us to an empowered state. We are not alone, our issues are not unique, and there is a solution to be found here as Jacquie bravely shares in her journey.

Patricia Meier

Reiki Master, Sound Healer, Hypnotist & Author

Balogh, as an advanced hypnotherapist, provides guidance and encouragement while she shows healers the way out from under "energy vampires" toward body and spirit harmony. This book also offers valuable information for caregivers who may forget that they, too, need to put themselves first while caring for others.

Annette Bower

Author

This is an excellent read for those looking to have a deeper understanding of the challenges they are facing within the body, mind and soul through their spiritual journey. Jacquie takes it one step further and shows us the light through it.

Tracy Roy

I like the idea of giving, not by being ultra-sympathetic and loading ourselves down with other people's burdens but by being whole in ourselves and vibrating at a higher energy level so that we bring people up to us rather than letting them drag us down to them. This book has something to offer everyone, because everyone knows what it feels like to be drained, to want to give, even to need to give, but having nothing left in the tank to give. Jacquie's book offers hope—good, practical hope—that it doesn't have to be this way.

Mary Balogh
Historical Novelist

This book is very well written, and easy to read. It will take you through the authors story of healing with hypnosis. This book is amazing for anyone struggling with burnout, and desires to heal themselves so they can help others. I love Jacquie's quotes and will be using many of them in my own practice. Very worth your time to read.

Gina Strole
Medium and Author of *FEAR BREAKTHROUGH - A Medium's Journey to Embracing Spirit*

Jacquie's book is a very accurate account of the experiences and exhaustion healers and therapists go through on the journey of healing others and themselves. She has great practical advice and tools to help you balance and guard your energy.

Cheryl Tessari
Certified Hypnotherapist, Reiki Master, Medium

THE
BURNED-OUT
HEALER

A Path to Trauma Release &
Reconnection to SELF

JACQUIE BALOGH

Wood Dragon Books

First Published 2020

Copyright © 2020 by Jacquie Balogh

Wood Dragon Books, PO Box 429, Mossbank, SK SOH 3GO

www.wooddragonbooks.com

ISBN: 978-1-989078-23-5

Cover Design: Callum Jagger

Author Photo: Jodi O Photography, Calgary, AB, Canada

For Tony

who has held my hand and my heart
through this journey
I'm your crazy forever
With all my love

For my Mum
who gave me the best advice
Just Start Writing
With all of my love and gratitude

TABLE OF CONTENTS

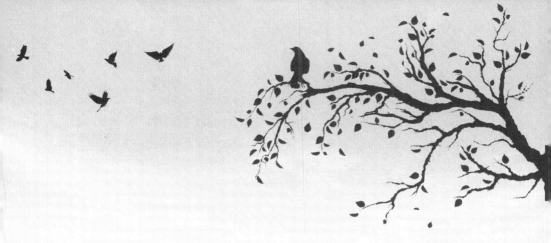

Introduction

Many of us wish that we could rewrite the story of our lives. As a spiritual worker and healer, I have had many times in my life when I wished that I could start again—rewrite the story that was playing out. When working to the healing of others, I found myself energetically and physically exhausted and burned out. This was my problem and, as I came to find out, the problem for many others who, like me, were working in the world of energy work and healing. Working with others no longer felt right. Rather than feeling rewarding, at the end of the day, it was draining.

How could I continue to work in my passion—my life's calling—without feeling constantly exhausted and burned out?

I was presented with the opportunity to change my story during one of the most trying times in my life. Working through the darkness of my days and toward the light, I found a solution that worked wonders for me and allowed me to begin to write this new story for my life. Once I had found the solution, I felt compelled to share it with others. From this desire to help came the formation of my *Reconnection to SELF* model which I share through hypnosis with my clients and in the pages of this book.

1

Through my own journey using this model, I was able to *reconnect* and my life changed in such amazing ways. The exhaustion left me and was replaced with an awakening and clarity. Working with others started to feel right again. My connection to universal energies was strengthened and I was able to attain greater depths of healing for myself and for my clients.

Through the course of my own journey, I was able to establish a stronger connection with my universal guidance team—those forces that are not seen but are always looking out for my best interest. From this newly strengthened relationship, I discovered that I was able to channel information. Some of this information was just for me and some was meant to be shared with others. Because the work I do is done in the deeper recesses of the higher mind and because the higher mind is the connection between the individual and universal energy—I feel a need to dive a little deeper here and allow my connection to the universe to have her say.

One day, as I was doing some self-hypnosis work (which is something I am continually doing as part of my own healing), I decided to ask about universal energy and in particular how God fit into the mix. The information I received was profound. It allowed me to shift my own life in many ways, especially when working with clients.

Let me preface what is to follow with a couple of points:

First and foremost, your belief system is yours and I am not one to debate what is better or worse, real or imagined. Your version of God and whatever word you use to describe the deity that is God (be it God, Source, Spirit, Creator, or any other) is yours. Your beliefs are yours and I encourage you to stay within them if that is your comfort level. Alternately, if you are curious and seeking, I would encourage you to explore in the direction of your choosing. Live and let live.

Secondly, hypnosis, in and of itself, has absolutely no basis in religion or God. It is a tool that is utilized as a scientific modality by those trained in the art to allow for exploration by the client into the deeper recesses of the mind for the purposes of curiosity, release, healing and forgiveness.

The following information is loosely transcribed from a session with me in a deeply hypnotic trance as I asked about God from the perspective of my connection to all universal energy. It may provide you some food for thought regarding your own life and belief systems.

These are the words of my connection.

"What is God?", I asked.

These are the words of my connection.

"We say that God is a man who lived and walked the earth so many years ago and that he had magical gifts that allowed him to heal the sick and to raise the dead and to bring words of peace to all those who chose to hear his words. It is a strong belief and it is a beautiful belief but God was never one man just as Jesus was never just one man. Stories have been told over time of the man who came to be known as the son of God walking the earth and doing his father's work in miracles. Neither were ever men in true human form (with supernatural abilities and powers); however, that is not to say that God never existed.

God, as humans know it to be, is a powerful energy.

All things are energy and all energy is connected and interconnected. Every man, woman, child; every beast and every other living thing is pure energy and all are connected. The word God, when spoken in human tongue, refers to one who is revered, one who is praised, one who leads. The human form of God appeared in the minds of man to allow for comprehension, to allow for a visual representation of the power of that energy.

God, as humans know it to be, is a powerful energy. There is no debate over this. All energy is connected and yet some energies are stronger, have specific purpose and yet remain only energy. God is such an energy, capable of great healing and great compassion and love for every living thing.

All energy is one energy and because of this all humans— all living things—are God! The energy that is God lives in all of us and is the source of what are known as the spiritual gifts. Examples include the gifts of healing, compassion, service, and vision. Every living being receives spiritual gifts when their soul combines to join their human host. Every day that humans choose to live in their sacredness and to share their gifts with others is a day that God energy shines within them.

Every day that humans choose to live in their sacredness and to share their gifts with others is a day that God energy shines within them.

It is amusing to those of us who have never been human to watch humans put things into categories: God, Devil, Good, Evil, Negative, Positive. It is as though humans need to live by category for their very survival. Energy is energy. It is that simple. It is not categorical. Where the human thought goes, the energy follows. If the human is living in suffering, they are in denial of their God energy and the blame falls on evil or negative

Energy is energy. It is that simple.

happenings. If the human is living in harmony, they are in balance and rejoicing in the goodness and positivity of their lives. There is no blame when times are good.

Who is God? God energy is neither male nor female, it is simply pure energy. God is in every human; God is in every living thing. Even the atheist human or the human who would give God another name is all one and all contain the God energy that is abundant as a universal source.

> *God energy is neither male nor female, it is simply pure energy. God is in every human; God is in every living thing.*

And yet, because of the human need to complicate and categorize, they bunch up and they hate. Humans hate color, language, race, religion. They hate with an energy equal to or greater than that of God energy. If humans could realize the connections that they have to the very fiber of their beings and to work collectively in their spiritual gifts, supporting, loving and connecting with each other… which is how it was supposed to have been… except that humans want choice, a basic human need. Humans want to decide and override the very energy—God energy—that they have built their hate around for untold centuries.

When you fall to your knees and you pray in times of crisis, when you stand in silent prayer wishing for better, for more, for change, you are praying to God energy and so you are praying to yourself and to all the world around you. The answers you are seeking are located within you as God energy and (because all energy is connected) within those around you who may rise and answer your call with their own God energy. Every human is equipped with the answers that they pray for every day. What

Every human is equipped with the answers that they pray for every day.

they don't realize is that they are never alone in the answers to their prayers.

Can you get silent? Can you delve deep enough within yourself to hear the answer when you, as God energy, answer your own prayer request? This is when there is the greatest disconnection from God energy. Humans ask for help and then they talk and talk and talk. They don't listen to themselves, see the dreams, or feel the God energy as it tries to guide them. Humans always choose to do things the hard-human way. Humans listen to reply and they never really listen to hear. God energy lives in every human and God energy speaks softly in the deepest silences. If you are brought to your knees and beg for the answer that will give you peace, will you stop and listen?"

When I emerged from this particular trance, I had a brand-new perspective and understanding and a deep sense of gratitude. I had been working on reconnection within myself and I was conflicted about where my gifts had come from and why they were so painful at times to work with. My gifts were my passion for helping and healing others, yet I was so exhausted and burned out that at times I had tried to quit—to run away from these gifts that felt like anything but.

What an amazing feeling of comfort it is to know that we are never, ever alone.

Understanding that God energy runs within me, as it does with every other human being on earth, made it much easier to understand how to work with energies—mine and others—in a way that honored and protected both parties. I was given the reassurance that all of the answers we are seeking, whether they are simple or complex, are sitting inside of us just waiting to be accessed.

God is me and I am God—as is every other human being on earth. What an amazing feeling of comfort it is to know that we are never, ever alone—that our purpose is love and connection in the spiritual gifts we were given to share with others.

How often have you heard someone, or perhaps even yourself say, "Karma will get them"? One evening, when I was doing self-hypnosis, I asked the question, "What is the difference between karma and trauma?" The following is the answer to my question

> *Trauma can be something as small as the sting of a bee or as significant as a near death experience.*

from the perspective of my connection to all universal energy. The answer may surprise you.

Again, these are the words of my connection.

"Karma and trauma are connected together like the weave of a spider's web.

Trauma occurs as a result of an event that causes a shift right down to the cellular level of a human. Trauma can be something as small as the sting of a bee or as significant as a near death experience. It anchors a part of us to the place and instant of impact. From that point, an idea is formed in the conscious mind of the human about how to feel and react each time something similar happens. Unless the trauma is dealt with at the deepest level of the self and released, it will continue to fester like an infected wound, growing larger and more traumatic as time passes. Many humans have lived lifetimes of the same trauma because they ignore the signals that the trauma is giving to release it. They instead think that each time something goes wrong, it is only a cruel reminder of the past event and they add another brick to their precarious wall of protection.

Unless trauma is dealt with at the deepest level of the self and released, it will continue to fester like an infected wound.

Many humans have no idea that there are those amongst them who have the gifts required to heal the wound, allowing the trauma to be released.

This is the nature of trauma.

Karma is the energetic recording of all traumas experienced in a single lifetime.

Karma starts at the moment of birth and stops at the moment of death of the human. Karma is the energetic recording of all traumas experienced in a single lifetime. It is also a recording of the release of any traumas in a lifetime. Some karmas are heavily laden with trauma and some are lighter. All karma can be lightened—simply by releasing trauma.

In this way, karma can be considered to be both good and bad. When a soul is at the point of choosing a life, it chooses a karma that requires attention. The soul then combines with the exact human body to live out all of the traumas of that karma in the hope that there will be the opportunity for the choice to release the traumas. The life of the human is largely dependent on their ability to remain in connection and communication with the soul and to be able to recognize that trauma can be released. A heavy and hard life generally means that trauma is still present and may even have been added to. A satisfactory, successful life means that traumas have been released.

There is a level of lifetime attainment that the rare few reach. This is a place of enlightenment (with the core beliefs of happiness, reason, nature, progress, and liberty) where all past traumas and karmas have been released. This is rare and so we will delve no further.

Regardless, at the end of almost every life there will be karma. Whether it is light or heavy is completely dependent on how much trauma was released and how much was picked up.

When humans wish for karma to befall another because of the state of their own existence and the human need to blame another, what actually happens is that the wisher adds to their own trauma. The other is living in their karma and is completely unaffected by another's wish that "karma" would befall them.

Sometimes an extraordinary human can and will overcome all of the trauma in their karma from a past lifetime. At that point, they are then allowed the opportunity to erase that karma completely from the record, so to speak. This is done at the point of creation where all souls choose. Once all of the trauma in a karma has been released, that karma ceases to exist."

Again, I was provided with a new perspective—one I certainly had never entertained. The idea that every single lifetime lived is a karma, and trauma is what is recorded—whether added to or released from—was very intriguing to me. It allowed me to move forward my work in *reconnection to SELF* at the deepest level. It allowed me to know the key importance as to why releasing trauma is so vital in living each lifetime to the fullest potential and to understand how karma plays such a vital role.

Having a deeper understanding about God energy—and the desire of the universe to allow me access to that energy any time I chose—allowed me to realize that every living thing is connected. If I was suffering, there were others around me who were as well. Perhaps I wasn't the only one exhausted and burned out.

Embracing God energy allowed me to get quiet with myself and to allow listening to take precedence over speaking. In this way, I was able to hear not only the problem at its root, but also the solution that had always been there. When it comes to others around me, I now know what I can contribute to their lives by way of healing without taking on their energies. God energy comes from within, and I had a means of guiding people to the point of listening to themselves. My gifts, which had once seemed anything but, became my strength when working with others' energies.

It is trauma that disconnects us from ourselves.

Knowing the difference between trauma and karma gave me a very simple model to work within. Understanding came when I realized that it is trauma that disconnects us from ourselves and that every trauma is added to the karma of a lifetime. When trauma is addressed and released, karma is lightened. Translation: When I face my problems and resolve them, they are no longer charged emotionally or physically and therefore are no longer harmful to my existence.

You can choose to use this information however you wish. At the very least, my sincere hope is that it has given you a fresh perspective about God, karma and trauma and where they fit into your own life and belief system.

Where do you see yourself now as you begin the journey that this book has intended for you?

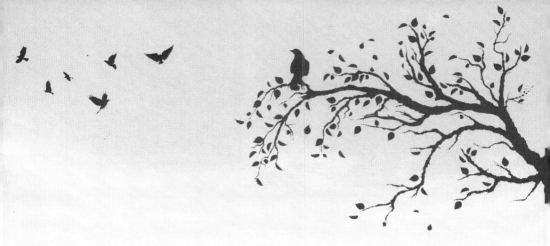

The Problem

I'm so very happy that you are here. You are a healer or energy worker—perhaps both. Whether that journey is a personal one or if it is your profession, this book and its story have found you for a reason. Throughout the course of this book, I will be referring to both healer and energy worker.

By now you've realized that there is a problem. You have been living a certain way, in a certain pattern of habits and beliefs—and they are not really working for you. You feel lost, disconnected, numb—living on auto pilot through most of your days. Maybe you can pinpoint the exact moment that you began to live this way—or maybe not. Regardless, you have come to the solid realization that something is not right and it needs to change. Perhaps you have tried to solve your problem—talking it out, thinking it out, willing yourself to change how you feel or act. Nothing has worked-otherwise you wouldn't be here right now.

As a healer and energy worker, you know that feeling of being compelled to do your work. After all, it is your passion, right? If it wasn't, it probably wouldn't be nagging at you constantly—even when you feel like you have nothing left to give. At the same time, you may feel that working in your passion is slowly pulling you apart. You are constantly giving pieces of yourself to others, but you aren't getting those pieces back in the "in-between" when you should be resting and recharging.

You ask yourself, *"Why do I feel so tired, so exhausted all the time? How can something that is supposed to be for the good of others make me feel so bad?"*

The emotional upheaval of your work is causing you to be tired, short tempered, and eventually—resentful.

You wish you knew the answer. You are an energy worker—a healer. How could you possibly stop giving to others what they need because this—*this very work that is exhausting you*—is who you are at your core?

So, you do know the answer to this problem, but the answer makes no sense.

You may find yourself eventually working on autopilot, moving through your daily activities like a robot because to expend additional energy would be the last straw. The emotional upheaval of your work and the needs of your clients weigh heavily on you, causing you to be tired, short-tempered and eventually—resentful.

Additionally, you may find yourself avoiding certain activities or events because you feel like you just can't face or take on any more energy. The grocery store is a landmine of people's energy that you pick up and carry home like unwanted groceries. Time spent with certain friends or family members leaves you feeling like you need to run and hide—you are in no position to want to feel all of their stuff. Because most family and friends know what you do, the underlying expectation is always that you are going to *just give them a little something*. They feel so much better after an emotional tune-up, while you sink further into exhaustion and resentment.

Yet, when someone calls for your help, for your time, for your energy, you are compelled to help them because that is just what you do. It is your gift and your purpose and to ignore it is completely impossible. So, you go and do what you can, absorbing all sorts of energies and

You are living in a chronically exhausted state and can't navigate your way out.

emotions. When you are done, you convince yourself that it is a *good exhaustion* because you have made someone else's life better in some way and that justifies you feeling this way. Deep down inside though, you know that this is not okay. You are exhausted. Even though others now feel better, you do not. And *that* is really *not* okay.

The problem is this: over time you have come to feel like hiding—like shutting off not only your passion but many other areas of your life as well. You don't have anything left to give, even to yourself. You are living in a chronically exhausted state and can't navigate your way out.

This is typically the outcome for those of us who are new to the world of healing and energy work. I understand this way of thinking very well, as I was once there too. Healers want to help and heal the world. In doing so, we fulfill our passion and our gift of service to others—without a thought or a care for ourselves. What

In living our passion to help and heal, we can completely forget that we need as much as we give.

we often forget to think about is that every exchange of energy comes at a price.

What about us? What about our own help and healing? In living our passion to help and heal and in sharing that gift of sensitivity and service to others, we can completely forget that we need as much as we give—more most of the time. This thought brings guilt and shame followed by the feeling that we are being selfish. After all, is it not wrong to want for ourselves if it takes away from what we give to others?

This vicious cycle of helping others, experiencing exhaustion, and then feeling shame begs the questions: Whose fault is it that we don't take the time to give to ourselves? Who is responsible for maintaining the protection of our own energies as healers and energy workers?

Of course, the answer is in the mirror.

How often do you put yourself and your needs first when it might mean saying "no" to another? Is it selfish to want to put yourself first? That is not the servant's heart, is it?

We tell ourselves that we are here to serve others and our own stuff can and will wait.

I would venture to guess that if you are reading this, you can honestly say that it is rare that you spend a great deal of time on self-care or spiritual hygiene—taking care of and protecting your own energies. I would also be willing to bet that you may be coming close to the point of wondering what you did to deserve this exhausting outcome.

Why can't you put yourself and your needs first? Because to do so, in your mind, would be the utmost in selfishness and self-absorption and that is not the way of a healer and energy worker. We tell ourselves that we are here to serve others and our own stuff can and will wait. *What a totally maddening thought.*

Have you ever thought of yourself as nothing or invisible? When we are tired and when we are resentful, we tend to ask the questions, "*Why me?*" and "*Why can't others see that I am not in the mood to help today?*"

These questions can lead to the bigger question, "*Am I completely unnoticed?*" Because of the exhaustion, there are times when we tend to want to blame the outside world and its influences for our lot instead of looking squarely in the mirror at the problem.

You've probably wondered who is at fault. After all, you are doing good work, but *you* are the one left suffering. You're asking yourself on a daily basis, "*Why can't I just feel better?*" and strangely enough, the answer just isn't coming forward.

If this problem of yours has reached its boiling point, you may have even thought about quitting. Taking on the energies and emotions of others is draining, exhausting and really not as rewarding as you thought it might be. Some days it would be just so easy to quit and walk away. Let someone else help and heal the world while you hide and lick your own wounds. Just let it all go. It would make life so much easier to just not feel this way—to simply not care.

Or would it?

When we came into this world, our soul chose to live out certain life experiences. It was given this body, this work of perfection, in order to live out all of those experiences. Along with the choice of body, the soul was equipped with a unique and specific set of spiritual gifts and skills to allow it to live out those experiences.

The soul is pure and requires very little—it is not human, as we experience life. So, "the problem" begins when human emotions get in the way. Why on earth would we want to feel everything an empath feels? Why on earth would we want to take on energies that are not our own so that another can experience relief from their suffering?

The answer is simple and complex. We do it because it is what we were put here to do. Our lives are less about the human experience and more about the soul experience. As humans, we are dragged along and compelled to do the work. We do it even though we are exhausted, both energetically and physically, and there is no end in sight to the work that still needs to be done!

Maybe it is the fault of our soul? Maybe we can place the blame squarely on the very energy that lives within us? But then, the soul chose this body for good reasons and because the soul is of pure energy, it couldn't have chosen wrong, right?

Well then, if it is not the fault of the soul, it has to be our own humanness that is the problem. If our souls are pure and don't make mistakes, then it has to be our own humanness that is the cause of "the problem". Maybe we're too empathic. Maybe we need to take more control of the situation. Maybe we need to override the voice in our head that is telling us that this is as good as it gets. Maybe our willpower needs to be strengthened. What it boils down to is that we just want to feel better and at this point, we don't even care how that happens. We just know it needs to happen now—before we become completely disconnected from our entire life!

What is it costing to continue down this path in this way? By now, you know that there is a problem. If you dive into that problem, you will see patterns, beliefs and habits that have been created as crutches to help you cope. These take on characteristics that are debilitating, or unmotivating at best. You may notice a lack of

Isolation exists in your life because it makes it easier to avoid people, places and situations than to face your problem head-on.

personal care, have an alarming number of physical ailments, and a trail of excuses, cancelled appointments and missed opportunities. It's costing you and it doesn't need to.

If you dive really deep, you may notice that the isolation exists in your life because it makes it easier to shut off and avoid people, places and situations rather than to face your problem head-on.

You don't receive joy from the things you once did. A simple cup of coffee at your favorite coffee shop is impossible as it turns into an energetic mine field from those around you. Conversations with family and friends always seem to spiral down into them wanting something from you. Every activity seems to require an expenditure of energy that you just don't have.

You bargain with yourself in an attempt to convince yourself that you can and will keep your healing work and energy exchanges completely separate from your personal life. Unfortunately, willpower alone hasn't made that a reality in the past—you can't separate one from the other because it is all you. You hold onto a faint hope that things will change, but you know that you are only setting yourself up for failure once again.

If this problem isn't solved soon, you may even consider stopping healing and energy work altogether, walking away from the gifts you were given to share with the world, knowing full well that the cost of giving up would be misery because this work is your passion and your calling. Think about it... what would it cost you to never again help or heal?

I have been exactly where you are. I know all about the brain fog, the exhaustion, and the deep desire to quit. I know that feeling of wanting to let go, thinking that it would be so much easier to let someone else deal with the emotional stuff of others. And I know what it cost when I tried—and failed—to quit.

I knew I had to come up with another way. I knew that quitting was not a solution and I knew that I did not want to continue to live the way I was. I knew that I had to figure out a way to protect myself from the energies I was working with while living out my passion. I knew I had to find a balance between my work and myself.

The next chapter is my story. I am honored to share it with you and to offer you hope, compassion, understanding, and a light at the end of your tunnel.

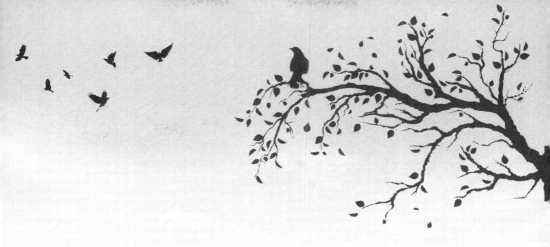

My Journey

From as far back as I can remember, I knew that I was different—that I had the ability to help people in special ways. I had a special knack for reading people, for knowing things about them that I really had no realistic way of knowing. I was able to see things around them such as auras and visitors from another realm. I was able to decipher what those things meant and I was able to help people along their journey just by sharing this knowledge with them.

As I grew into adulthood, I knew that I needed to help people and so, as any logical human being would do, I pursued a career that would involve helping others. I initially chose a career in the healthcare field. I became a licensed practical nurse and I enjoyed a wonderful fifteen-year career before becoming disillusioned with a system that focused more on bureaucracy than healing. As I walked away from that career, I found myself feeling like a fish out of water. What would I do now? I wanted to work with people using my gifts for healing but I did not want to work within a system that did not align with my own vision and goals.

I trained and read about various energetic pursuits, incorporating my knowledge into my own healing and energy work as I went along. Reiki, tarot, mediumship and psychic work, access bars, coaching, and finally—hypnotherapy. I loved the charge I got out of working with energy. It gave me great satisfaction when I worked with others and knew that I was truly helping them clear their own paths of whatever had been holding them back.

The problem was that even though I thoroughly enjoyed working in this passion of mine, I was living in a chronic state of exhaustion and brain fog. I was losing interest in other areas of my life because I had nothing left to give of myself.

Eventually, I decided to separate the passion from the person and, for a time, I believed I had accomplished this separation. I thought of my healing and energy work as a separate part of my life. I would go out, do what work was asked, and then I would step back into my human existence again. It was separate, two parts of the same being. It never occurred to me that my work had to be in rhythm with my entire being.

In the middle of a July night in 2017, I woke up from what I thought was a horrible dream. In the dream, I was upside down in a vehicle trapped in the dark and underwater—one of my greatest fears. I knew in the dream that I had to get out. The problem was not getting out of the seatbelt, it was getting out of a car that was upside down in the water and in complete darkness. In the deafening silence of the dream, I was terrified and paralyzed—full of confusion. I did what I imagine any normal human being would do in that situation... I woke up.

The dream was over, but the nightmare was just beginning.

In the ensuing moments, I remember coming awake very briefly; a very strange feeling taking hold of me. The next memory I have is explaining in a very panicked way to my husband that I thought I had just had a seizure. There had been a short period of time between waking up and actually being able to speak to him—a period of time that I have no memory of at all.

Just when I thought maybe it was a part of the dream, I was hit with another seizure. This continued again and again—voids in memory and loss of muscular control—over the course of the rest of the night as my terrified husband could only comfort me with his words, letting me know that I was not alone. Eventually, I ended up in an ambulance on my way to the emergency room. I had no idea or frame of reference for the way I was feeling.

The seizures were very real. I did not have the markers for epilepsy, and I was diagnosed with PNES or Psychogenic Non-epileptic Seizure Disorder. PNES is the cause of psychological factors that present

This is the awakening and conjunction of your human life and your journey with spirit.

themselves in the form of seizures. These factors go far beyond the normal symptoms of anxiety and even beyond panic attacks. They cause seizure activity and fully shut down the body, often multiple times within minutes. The diagnosis was a relief, the treatment options were not.

I remember the day that I was diagnosed and the suggestion that I should book an appointment with a psychiatrist. I very clearly remember something inside of me crying out that psychiatry and medications weren't the way to deal with this. The voice inside of me was screaming loud and clear, "*This requires deep reflection. This requires you to release what is holding you stuck to the floor. This is the awakening and conjunction of your human life and your journey with spirit. This requires more than talking and medicating. This requires focus and determination and decision making unlike anything else you have ever encountered before. Make the decision now."*

How does one ignore the voice? Does one even try to ignore the voice? Faced with a complete lack of what I considered viable options, and completely terrified, I chose very quickly to listen to that voice.

After discussion with my physician, I walked out of his office and into an idea—I would use hypnosis as the medium to sort out the cause of my own problem.

Could I heal myself? Could I heal what needed to be healed in order to rid myself of this condition? As a healer, medium and hypnotherapist, I knew that the answers were "yes" and so I set out to begin the process of awakening within myself. I contacted a trusted mentor and friend who was one of the most talented hypnotherapists I knew and together we began the work of releasing the stuff that was holding me stuck to the floor in order to make room for the awakening process to take shape within me—or as I visualized it, a rising out of the ashes.

I am one being and how I do one thing was how I do all things.

Being a healer is a passion for me and my best process for helping others to heal is hypnosis. I have been a healer as far back as I can remember both in this lifetime and in what I believe to be many past lifetimes as well. But what I hadn't realized was that I had been operating with a huge disconnect—healing is my passion but life was necessary to live that passion. I am one being and how I did one thing was how I did all things.

As a healer, I would throw myself into my energy work with all the passion I could muster and then I would find myself exhausted and tired. Eventually, other parts of my life became neglected and off-balance because of this exhaustion. I wasn't acknowledging or embracing the synthesis of my life and the seizures were the eventual sum total of my soul and physical body not wanting that imbalance any longer. The seizures were brought to me to literally drop me to my knees so that I would stop and breathe; so that I could choose to get back into balance. They were a pattern interrupt, if you will, allowing me the opportunity to realize the imbalance and then to choose to work and live in synthesis.

> *We are taught that surrender translates to loss of control. Surrender is the closest thing to control that we do have.*

Now you may think that this was a simple process and you would be both right and wrong. Hypnotherapy is a wily art and a creative teacher. In hypnotherapy, anything and everything is possible through simple choice. In my case, there was an element of letting go of control that needed to take place, as well as surrender to the idea that what I was doing wasn't working. As humans, we have a need to control as we feel it is the only thing we have. In reality, there is no such thing as control. As humans, we are taught that surrender translates to loss of control and weakness; however, surrender is the closest thing to control that we do have.

25

When I realized that I had control over nothing and that surrender meant moving *into* what was truly best for me, I could begin to heal. It was that simple.

Through the process of doing my personal work in hypnotherapy, I chose to give up control of my life and my mind to my higher self. I began the work of surrendering based on the idea that I knew what was best for me. I gave up trying to control all of the outcomes, the fear that I had over losing control, and the fury that I had over feeling exhausted and burned out all the time.

I was curious about what was causing the issues that I was having in my life. How could I work within myself to change things for the best for me in my work as a healer and in living my life? In the end, it was this curiosity that caused the most significant shift and the most profound change.

Working with a great mentor and friend creates a very comfortable feeling of trust and support. Having someone to work with who you have built trust and rapport with, someone who will hold that space for you, makes the work so much easier.

When we use the term *"holding space for another"*, we literally mean sitting in silence while another works through their issues and moves toward solution. It means being energetically invested in the outcomes of another and doing what is necessary to clear the path for the release of the bad stuff and the transformation to the good stuff. It is investing in another with the clear understanding that gains are of no consequence to the one holding space, save a positive outcome for the client. It means not interfering with the process with one's own judgements.

Holding space for another means that there is very clear knowledge that growth of any kind, but especially spiritual growth, as was the case with me, never happens easily and never at times of rest. It literally happens in the midst of hell—when one is struggling, frustrated, angry, fearful, invisible, horrified, exhausted, seizing—and the only one capable of making a different choice is the one going through it.

Happily, I can say that my mentor gave me all the time and space that I needed then and now to work through my own stuff and to come to my own realizations. She gave me the gift of space held just for me and time to shift and change and to choose a better way. I found the ability to choose to let go of control and to surrender to what is best for me. I developed a real trust with myself and with my higher mind. There are times when I am reminded, by way of small seizures, that I am just hovering on the brink of stepping backwards into chaos. I, again, am allowed to choose the path of surrender. Most of all, I have found someone who truly understands how to hold space while standing on the outside in a supporting role as I continue to open and to grow.

> *Surrender requires completely trusting in one's self—that even when things seem to be falling apart, they are actually falling into a better place.*

It has not been an easy road. In the beginning, it was often messy and ugly because it was not easy for me to detach from the human need to control, or to learn to trust that there was a higher power looking out for me, ready to catch me as I fell out of the old and familiar and into the new and unknown. Surrender is the harder of the two as it requires completely trusting in oneself—that even when things seem to be falling apart, they are actually falling into a better place. Eventually, messy and ugly gave way to clarity, focus, and blessed peace and balance.

It became apparent to me that if I was experiencing this kind of emotional and spiritual rollercoaster as a healer and energy worker—disconnecting from my own deepest self—then surely there must be others out there experiencing the same thing. After facing the worst and choosing to do the work for myself, I experienced such profound positive gains in my own life that I felt I needed to share this success story with others. The journey that I had been on was not only for me, but it was also a story begging to be shared. If only one person could experience that profound reconnection in their own life, then my story would be worth the telling.

The main problems for me were the exhaustion, the brain fog, the burnout; the energetic turmoil that I took on from others while working with them. This was my need to try to control the healing, which—of course—is completely impossible. When I let go of this need to control, I started to see myself in a totally different light. I was a person too and I deserved to work in my passion *and* have a life of my own.

In releasing that need to control, I came to see my clients in a different light as well. It became easy to let go of the need to control and to just hold space for them to feel their own feelings and to make their own choices. It became easy to allow their energetic mess to flow through and disperse. It was no longer my burden to shoulder. The idea that I gained nothing from their success, save their positive outcome, freed me from the need to give them what they wanted. I could simply allow them the time to surrender into what they already knew they needed all along and their choice to incorporate it. The idea of *holding space for another* gave me the realization that I am me and they are them and that I could choose to just allow whatever their choice was.

Through my own personal journey with hypnotherapy, I have learned the art of recognizing and releasing my need to control. I have further adopted a *go with the flow* attitude in all areas of my life, surrendering into things that are best for me. Releasing my need to control has brought me to a place of peace and connection with my deepest self and balance. I don't have seizures any longer as I have learned what I need to let go of, what I need to pay attention to in my own life—and that the lives of others are their own.

I have not only crafted the practice of working in my passion without allowing it to overwhelm other areas of my life, I am also creating better and better outcomes for myself and for my clients. There is a flow and a synthesis that has been created. Now instead of messy and ugly (because I no longer have the larger issues holding me stuck to the floor), life ebbs and flows and I choose the outcomes that I want for myself.

Gratefully, as a hypnotherapist, I get to share the opportunity of choice with my clients. I tell them that everything and anything is possible—which I believe to be true.

I help my clients realize that they know themselves best of all. When working on important issues in our lives, we often refer to the leading expert. In my case, that was me. In the case of my clients, I help them realize it is them. I hold the space for them as they choose to connect with their own higher mind and build trust with it. After that, they get to choose to experience their own reconnection to their deepest self.

What follows is the "idea" and the solution that I used to help and heal myself. I am hopeful that it will provide the insight and awareness that you are searching for on your own journey to healing.

Surrendering Control

Once I created a balance and a synthesis in my own life, I realized that I needed to share this knowledge with all healers and energy workers, no matter where they were on their journey. No one wants to walk around feeling broken, burned out, and disconnected from their own life. There was light at the end of the tunnel and I wanted to share that light.

Are you thinking that you are broken? That something is seriously wrong with you? How it's impossible to find balance in your life as you keep taking on more and more from others, leaving you exhausted and feeling like your brain is in the clouds? How do you find the balance in something you don't even fully understand?

> *No one wants to walk around feeling broken, burned out, and disconnected from their own life.*

It's simple… We are not broken; we don't need fixing. We are hurting, we need healing.

and energy workers need as much healing as they
others—if not more. Plain, simple and non-negotiable.
eed to be more important in our own lives than those we
here to serve.

I realize now that long before the seizures took hold of me,
I was suffering. I was always tired; and healing work depleted
any energy I did have. Healing work is my passion, however,
the energy working in it was literally killing me. My mind was a
jumble. I felt a disconnection from everyone and everything. I
just wanted to be left alone to try and rebuild my energies for
the next person who required my services.

> *Spiritual workers and healers need as much healing as they give to others—if not more.*

A few years before the seizures
began, I quit. I stopped doing any kind
of energy or healing work. I hid behind
a mask of indifference because I
was tired and I just wanted to get
through the day without feeling like I
needed to borrow tomorrow's store of energy to move forward.
Unfortunately, or so I believed at the time, I felt compelled to
return to my work once again. It was a part of me, and it needed
to be brought forth for others. This is the path of working within
one's gifts. There is no ignoring the calling for any long period
of time without upsetting the balance.

Even through the indifference, I was still exhausted. It took
as much energy to try and ignore my passion as it did to work
within it.

I finally saw the light at the end of the tunnel when I chose to
put myself and my needs first. I needed to make changes in my
entire life because energetically I was exhausted and others
areas of my life were quickly following suit. The seizures were,

in their own way, the light at the end of my own tunnel. They made me pause, make decisions, and make changes. They presented a choice to change an unfortunate situation into a fortunate one.

> *Working on ourselves is as hard or as easy as we choose to make it.*

Working on ourselves is as hard or as easy as we choose to make it. We rarely spend as much time working on ourselves as we should and often don't begin until we are faced with the reality that we no longer have a choice in the matter.

It is not until we decide that we are going to put ourself first in our life that profound change can happen. This means putting ourselves before our spouse, our kids, our career, our friends. ALL of it! We must come first. This means facing the harsh reality that our methods for trying not to feel exhausted and disconnected have failed up until now. It means that right now, in this moment, we get to choose whether or not we are ready to stop paying the price for our passion. It means choosing a future that can be more of the same—or profoundly better.

For me, it was an easy decision. I felt like I had nothing left to give myself and definitely nothing left to give others. I knew that I didn't want to carry on living my life in the same painful way that I had been. I wanted the seizures to stop and that meant focusing all of my time and attention on myself. Ironically, and importantly, one of the first things that I worked on was the dual guilt of putting myself first and *not* putting myself first. I was still trying to work with clients while working on myself and I needed to find a balance between them and me. At first, I struggled with the guilt of shifting my focus to me, and then I surrendered.

And, when I did, magic started to happen.

Reprogramming the mind takes everything we believe and turns it upside down and sideways. The potential of the human mind to expand and to change is nothing short of amazing.

The conscious mind is the mind that lives in the everyday. It uses our programming as a roadmap to protect us in the world we live in and our perception of it. However, as with every yin, there is a yang. The conscious mind is also our fiercest critic. It is the little voice you hear, better known as *ego*, that tells you not to step outside of your safe zone, that you are not worthy, that you shouldn't expect more out of life, that there is no room for growth or change, that this is how you should feel. Your ego is a voice that says that as long as everything stays the same, everything will be fine—even if you're physically exhausted.

Willpower is our conscious effort to silence the voice of the ego.

Read that last sentence again. Do you notice how *ego* uses its voice to accost you from within?

It is ego that creates what we know as willpower. Willpower is our conscious effort to silence the voice of the ego. It is our conscious attempt to change at the most superficial level of the mind. Willpower is one of our weakest lines of defense. It rarely works because it is constructed within the parameters of the ego. When those parameters are tested, ego will take the path of least resistance, resorting back to what has always been the status quo. That is why so many times, no matter how hard we fight against the voice of ego, willpower eventually fails us.

So how do we reprogram the mind? How do we reprogram everything we have always lived in order to get to something better? Where do you go when you don't know where to go?

You go to the expert, my friend—you.

By sinking deeper into the mind, we can get past the conscious mind and into the wise and all-knowing subconscious mind. The subconscious mind is our literal mind. It records every single detail of everything we have ever experienced. It is always awake and alert even when we are asleep.

Sometimes the subconscious mind is so eager to get our attention that it speaks to us in dreams. Have you ever had a dream that was so vivid and so real that you remembered every detail? Generally, it is a dream about a change or something that you have been thinking about for a while. These dreams often make a great deal of sense. This is your subconscious mind communicating with you and attempting to give you the answers you've been looking for.

The subconscious mind controls approximately ninety-five percent of our lives and is referred to as the "feeling mind," as this is where our emotions are stored. It is many times stronger than the conscious mind and it has the power to stop the ego and its weak willpower in its tracks, opening the mind further to explore much more powerful and impactful outcomes holistically.

To reprogram the mind, the subconscious needs to be accessed. There, all permanent change takes place. There is no willpower, there is only the literal in the subconscious. This means

> *Hypnosis is one of the easiest and most effective ways to bypass the conscious mind and to deeply access the subconscious mind.*

that when a suggestion for change is made, the subconscious takes it at face value and makes the change in the areas of your life that it needs to. Out with the old thought and in with the new.

Hypnosis is one of the easiest and most effective ways to bypass the conscious mind and to deeply access the subconscious mind.

Being able to work in your passion and serve others is possible without energetically exhausting your own life force.

When we live in ego—only on the outside of ourselves—we shut the color out of our lives. It is as if we only see black and white, limiting the beauty of connection and growth. But when we choose to go deeper, accessing our subconscious mind, we release all of the intense colors of life and what is possible from within. Imagine the kaleidoscope that you could create when using all of the colors in your own life!

Making permanent positive change in your life creates a connection that allows for peace and balance rather than exhaustion and disconnection. Being able to work in your passion and serve others is possible without energetically exhausting your own life force.

Really understanding the power of putting myself first and taking care of my energy allows me to work within my passion as a healer, yet not take on and hold onto the energies of others. It is about respecting my own boundaries and living within them. Most importantly, it is about the deep connection with myself and honoring that balance in all areas of my life.

In the following chapters, I will be sharing with you the model that brought me back to myself and allowed me to be able to find the balance between working in my passion and living my daily life.

The model is simply called *Reconnection to SELF* because, in very simple terms, it is a process that leads you from where you are now to plugging into and fine-tuning the balance within yourself and then maintaining that balance.

I'll be diving deep to explore the little-known opportunities of working with the subconscious mind. With clearly laid out objectives and outcomes, the world is yours to own as you choose to do the work that is most important for you.

Healing is an inside job. In the following chapters, you will gain insights into trauma at its core and how the loss of connection to SELF is the culprit, how approaching a problem holistically allows for major insights into some of the underlying and often ignored causes, and how profoundly this disconnection is affecting your health and wellbeing. You will gain further insight into reprogramming and why it is so important that this reprogramming be done at the subconscious level of the mind. You will learn about everyday maintenance that will keep you moving in the direction you want to be moving in and away from where you are now.

Think about your passions, your relationships, your everyday life. What needs attention right now? What needs to be nourished? My hope is that you will begin to see yourself, your problem, and the answers you are seeking for yourself through the framework of the *Reconnection to SELF* model.

If YOU have a problem… YOU are your solution.

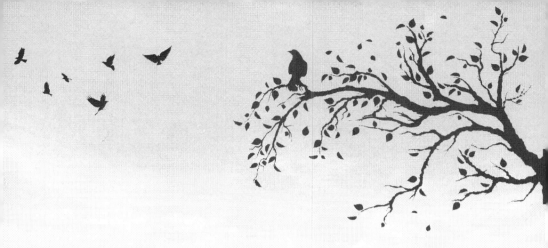

Understanding Trauma

Trauma is caused when we have a problem. Trauma causes changes in us. Whether or not those are good changes or bad changes, you can rest assured that if you have experienced trauma, you have changed.

You were probably attracted to this book because you have suffered long enough and because that suffering has changed you. You have realized that there is a problem and that it is no longer acceptable to either cope or live with it. You have experienced a trauma or multiple traumas that have compounded to the point of being seriously uncomfortable, even unbearable. That pain has led you here—to a solution that sticks.

Thinking about the work that you do as a healer and energy worker, I can only assume that you have experienced the weight of energetic exhaustion, brain fog, burnout, a feeling of disconnection from the rest of your life—and it has reached a point where you are no longer willing to live this way.

How often can you remember feeling tired or fatigued after working with energy? As you think back, you will start to gain an understanding of the gravity of what you have been carrying and of just how much suffering you've endured in the name of working in your passion. Some may be able to trace this feeling back as far as childhood. These gifts, after all, are lifelong.

When we think of trauma, we tend to think of huge, massive, life-altering events.

When I finally realized the true gravity and immensity of the trauma that I had been living with, I was devastated. I was angry, sad, and fearful for the damage that I had done to myself. Most importantly, I was resigned and willing to discover what it would be like to no longer have to carry the result of all of that trauma around with me. Eventually, I turned hopeful… and then I surrendered into becoming someone I could recognize once again. I embraced true, transformative change.

When the word trauma is used, we often think of emergency rooms, messy and unorganized from the rushing of staff to save a life. The visual is often one of panic and chaos. When we think of trauma in terms of an assault on our own person, we tend to think of huge, massive, life-altering events. You have heard others and perhaps even your own voice say, *"That experience has changed me for life"* or *"I will never be the same again"*. If you think back through the course of your life, you can pick out the events that were the most traumatic. Or sometimes they were so damaging and impactful that you have blocked the memory of them altogether.

But what about the small stuff? The everyday mundane things that begin to build into bigger things? Think about the healing work that you do. If you are in the service of others, how often have you felt sick, tired, exhausted, or distracted after a day of work? How often do you walk away from your work feeling that, at that moment, *you* are the one in need of healing? If you had taken the time to recognize those feelings and to deal with them appropriately with solid self-care, then that small stuff would have passed through and moved on, leaving you feeling balanced and energized once again.

However, if I am correct, you were called to this book and you are reading this information because the path of self-care and self-healing is not the path you have chosen to follow until now. Maybe you didn't realize that it was an option. Perhaps you felt like you were being selfish because taking the time to put yourself first meant everyone else came second. Or you've thought that this is just how you are supposed to feel every day. There are a myriad of excuses and reasons that you tell yourself daily so that you can keep going.

> *Everything is connected energetically and so by allowing our energies to be completely depleted when working with others, other areas of our lives are depleted as well.*

The longer this has been allowed to go on in our life is as long as we have been causing trauma to build. As healers and energy workers, we know that everything is connected energetically and so by allowing our energies to be completely depleted when working with others, other areas of our lives are depleted as well. If you think about it in terms of energetic connection—how we do one thing is how we do all things. The trauma that has built over time is not only affecting our abilities as a healer and energy worker, it is affecting every other part of our life.

Trauma causes excuses, illness and disconnection. It makes you feel like there are pieces missing and because of that, you operate your life on autopilot, limping along, hoping that one day you will feel whole again.

Trauma is the reason you find yourself more and more wanting to crawl under a rock or hide in a corner. It is the reason you cancel appointments and bail on events. You may even send others out into the world to do the things that cause you suffering. In chapter one, I wrote that going to the grocery store could be like a land mine, where we walk around feeling exhausted in a brain fog, trying to get our groceries but picking up the energies of the others in the store. It's like taking home unwanted groceries. So, instead of doing it ourselves, we ask someone else to pick up the few things we need because we simply can't bear any more suffering.

Trauma can cause you to self-isolate.

You may find yourself purposely avoiding appointments or events with friends and family. You are tired and you can't face being around any kind of energy. This avoidance behavior may get to a point where friends and family no longer come around or invite you to events. The trauma has caused you to self-isolate. People are tired of your excuses, so they stop engaging. Initially, their response may seem like a blessing because all you want is a bit of peace and quiet. However, in social circles and society in general, this is also a curse. Sooner or later, you will have to face those people again which becomes a vicious competition of social obligations versus your own self-imposed and much needed social isolation.

But the excuses we give ourselves and others as to why we continue to work, even though it depletes us, come when we are called energetically or asked physically to help others. The reasons we do what we do, even at personal cost to ourselves, are abundant. They fall out of our mouths with a defiant force, convincing ourselves that working in our passions is not something that is optional. This is where the disconnect is clearly visible.

When we rationalize doing the thing that is causing us the most suffering, in our lives, we become completely disconnected from any sort of balance or harmony in our lives. We have tumbled into trauma.

> *Trauma is not a bad word; it is the word that we use to describe the depth of our pain.*

Trauma is not a bad word. It is the word that we use to describe the depth of our pain. When we are suffering so much that all areas of our lives are affected, that is trauma. The good news is that all we have to do is to ask for help. Trauma is perhaps the most misunderstood cause of human suffering, but it does not have to be this way.

What is your problem? What is it that is causing you to feel exhausted and burned out from doing the healing and energy work that you do?

By now you have realized that the way you have been living and feeling is no longer acceptable. There is another way to be and that comes on the other side of trauma—specifically, on the other side of dealing with that trauma.

This is an opportunity for you to start thinking back to when this all started and when it began to affect other areas of your life. Your passion is your pain at the moment because this is where you have experienced the most suffering. The healing work that you do leaves you feeling exhausted, and burned out, and those feelings have leaked into other areas of your life. Digging deeper, what exactly is it about your passion that causes the pain?

It is at the exact spot in your lifetime where trauma took place. Something happened and it caused a change in you. That moment in time is anchored at the energetic and cellular level of your being.

A physical anchor is a heavy thing that holds boats to ground; an emotional anchor is a heavy thing that holds us stuck to the floor—unable to move freely forward.

A physical anchor is a heavy thing that holds boats to ground. An emotional anchor is a heavy thing that holds us stuck to the floor—unable to move freely forward. It can span over this lifetime and into future lifetimes as well. Imagine the weight of all of your traumas that have not been dealt with in this and previous lifetimes. That is a phenomenal amount of weight.

Are you stuck to the floor—anchored?

When a trauma drops anchor in your life, it is the cause of fears, phobias, habits, and patterns that govern your life. Anchors are powerful things and their power is compounded when trauma is attached. The only way for a ship to sail is to become unstuck from the floor of the ocean by weighing anchor and releasing the hold on the sand.

In releasing trauma, your work begins by recognizing those trauma laden anchors that are holding you stuck to the floor.

The only way to break free of the effect of the anchor is to energetically raise it up and release the hold it has on you. This first step to healing is recognizing that trauma has taken place in your life and that it has changed you. It is what is causing the exhaustion, the burnout, and even the desire to quit working with energy. It is what has and will continue to cause chaos in all areas of your life unless you choose to face it head on and deal with it.

When we think about exhaustion, brain fog, burnout and how they affect our lives as a whole, we think about events, situations, or people outside of ourselves as the major contributing factors. In short, we look for someone other than ourselves to blame.

But what if these symptoms are all coming from within? What if we have dealt ourselves so much trauma and self-neglect that we have become disconnected from an important part of the very core of ourselves—a place called *SELF*?

Think about our lives in terms of a circuit board—a maze of wires, connections, and interconnections that keep machines running effectively. The *SELF* is like a circuit board that, when fully functional and working optimally, allows us to always be at our best in any given moment, to stand in our own personal power, and to speak our truth in an impactful way. The SELF is connected to our core, controlling connection and communication between our soul and our humanness (body and mind). When it is operating optimally, we are in complete balance within ourselves.

But what happens to a circuit board when one circuit goes haywire? The whole system stops working—or at least it goes into limp mode. What if our bodies are designed like this circuit board and that the real cause of our trauma is lack of connection and communication at the core?

There are no outside forces that can inflict emotional, mental or spiritual suffering on any single human.

What if all of your problems are coming from inside of you instead of from outside influences as you may have previously thought? *Perhaps the exhaustion and burnout that you are experiencing when working energetically in the world comes not from others, but as a direct result of self-neglect, lack of self-care and a malfunctioning circuit board in your SELF—causing chaos on the inside and manifesting itself in your outer world as exhaustion, burnout and disconnection.*

Are you the malfunctioning circuit in your own life—the one that, if connected properly, would weigh anchor on your traumas?

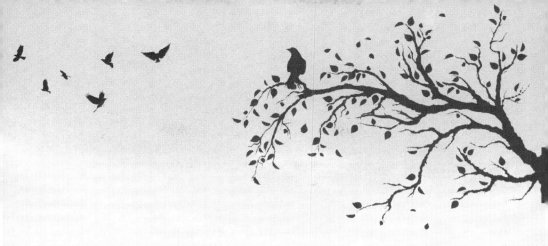

Expanding Perspective

The *SELF* is a place of love and connection that exists deep inside the body, mind, and soul and manifests in actions and emotional responses to the outside world. It works in conjunction with the core system in our bodies including the spirit, soul, the emotional heart, the upper brain (mind) and the lower brain (intuition or gut). When this core system is in balance—connection and communication are optimal—our *SELF* is in complete harmony.

For the purposes of understanding the *core system* further, the actual body encompasses body, mind and soul. When referring to *spirit*, this is a universal force outside of the actual body that has connection through the soul. Spirit may also be called by other names; universe, source, God (or other deities), or higher mind.

As with everything in life, there are strengths and weaknesses. One cannot exist without the other and this is true of all opposites.

Even the soul and our basic humanness are working in a yin and yang, balancing energies back and forth in order for the soul to live out its purpose—as was predetermined in spirit prior to incarnation—and the actual human body to provide the medium for those experiences.

When even one small glitch appears, the system begins to malfunction, falling into chaos and disconnection from *SELF*. This is known as trauma.

All human trauma stems from the internal world and lives deep in the mind. All trauma is self-inflicted. In saying this, I don't mean that as humans we go around looking to hurt ourselves. Bad things happen in the human world—we hear about them every day. What I mean is that when a trauma occurs, it is internalized by the individual and their story determines how they will act or react in the future as a result of this trauma.

Outside influence is often the cause that humans ascribe to a problem. It is why two people can experience the same event and react in completely different ways. However, we as humans have evolved over time enough to know that all suffering and resulting trauma stems from within.

The exhaustion you feel from picking up the energies of others when working with them is a classic example of the accumulation of trauma.

The conscious mind, or ego, would have us believe that the cause of our suffering is the result of something outside of us. It looks for faults and blame where there are none. There are no outside forces that can inflict emotional, mental or spiritual suffering on any single human.

It is the core system that interprets all things, but the human experience that lives them out. If human experience was removed from the equation, then there would be absolutely no effect on us—save physical—from outside influence as all feeling and emotion would be removed.

Much like an author records words on the pages of a book, through every moment of our lives including sleep, the subconscious

Your problem as you thought it was may not be your problem at all.

mind records facts and events as it sees, hears, smells and feels them—without judgement and without emotion. Some of these things are joyous, happy, triumphant events; things that make us humanly feel good about ourselves. Some of these things are the exact opposite—so dark, vile, and cruel—that a part of the mind actually blocks out the memory of the entire event—choosing only to let the memory resurface when one too many traumas are added to the original.

Whatever has been recorded dictates how we live in the world, just as the words recorded in a book tell us the story. All of our patterns, habits, fears, phobias come from the story of our

It is the sole purpose of the higher mind to eliminate the negative in order to make room for the positive.

lives. The traumas are woven into the story in intricate detail. Without knowledge or a depth of understanding, we live our lives based on the traumas we have suffered in the past. Without us realizing it, some of our traumas get larger and larger. Suffering compounds upon suffering, affecting us more as the trauma builds. The exhaustion you feel from picking up the energies of others when working with them is a classic example of the accumulation of trauma. Has that exhaustion not crept its way into all other areas of your life in some way, shape or form?

The *higher mind*, which is a branch of the subconscious mind and connected to all universal energy (spirit), knows how to resolve these traumas. It is the sole purpose of the higher mind to eliminate the negative in order to make room for the positive. Unfortunately, we are human, and as humans, we have choice; choice often leads us to choose to continue living in chaos. Humanness, and in particular, human emotion, is a messy business. But there is a path out of chaos.

As I mentioned earlier, when the core system is in balance, the human experience is wonderful. When we experience balance, we are also in harmony within the SELF.

There are nine key areas of the SELF that require balance in order to relieve suffering and to release trauma. In no particular order and equal in importance, they are:

- Self-Esteem
- Self-Confidence
- Self-Love
- Self-Worth
- Self-Image
- Self-Acceptance
- Self-Awareness
- Self-Actualization
- Self-Care

When these nine areas are balanced, it is easy for us to put ourselves first in our lives and for trauma to be released. It is easy to set goals and to expand on them for the future. When these areas are balanced, there is an inner homeostasis that settles through the core system and all areas of life improve becoming easier to manage-including our passion as healers and energy workers.

Loss of SELF in any of these key areas means that a trauma has taken place at some point in time, either in this lifetime or another. Some people are born into this world with a SELF that is not intact as a result of trauma from a past life. These traumas carry over from one life into another because they have yet to be resolved.

Welcome to this step in the *Reconnection to SELF* model. To quickly review, we spent some time defining what trauma is and how it shows up as disconnection from the deepest SELF. Next, we delved into the SELF and discovered that disconnection occurs with trauma.

> *You have an untapped wealth of knowledge about yourself locked up in the recesses of your mind.*

The first part of this step is about surrendering into the idea that your problem as you thought it was may not be your problem at all. All trauma comes from within and so your actual problem is not just skin deep, you are not just exhausted. You are in fact disconnected from the deepest core of you—the SELF that controls connection and communication between your soul and your humanness.

There are different levels of the mind and the deeper you go—moving out of humanness and into spiritual energy—the less emotional and personal things are. Because you now understand that your higher mind knows exactly how to fix this problem of yours, you may realize something profound. You have this untapped wealth of knowledge about yourself locked up in the recesses of your own mind.

You are the key to your own suffering. You are the key to releasing your own traumas. You are the key to reconnecting with that deepest part of the SELF and bringing about balance and harmony within your own core system.

All of this time, you have been walking around exhausted and burned out and ready to quit doing your healing and energy work. You've been searching for the answers that will give you peace and balance in your life. You have been looking to find a way to work in your passion while feeling protected from the energies of others. All this time you have been searching for the expert who will solve your problem. Isn't it a wonderful thing to realize that the expert you have been looking for… is you?

By now you realize what the problem is, how deeply it runs, and you realize where the problem is coming from. So now what do you do about it?

When I work with clients who conclude that they are disconnected from the *SELF*, I generally have one statement and question for them. It is simple, it is easy, and it is totally achievable.

You know what you don't want in your life, how you don't want to feel and how you don't want to act. So, what do you want instead?

> On the other side of trauma are connection and balance.

Once you have decided what you want instead, it is about setting goals and achieving them quickly, easily, efficiently and permanently. This involves setting goals, changing your mind, changing your lifestyle, changing the very fiber of your being—in short—self-healing.

This second part of this step is about building on your goals based on the importance of solving your problem. How badly do you want to change the story of your life? This is an important component of your success because as humans we are very patterned. We do what we've always done because it is what we know and because it keeps us safe. Change is not safe. It requires accepting that things cannot stay the same and stepping out of your comfort zone. On the other side of trauma are connection and balance. Can you let go of the chaos that the traumas have caused when that is all you have known?

What are your motivating factors for wanting and living permanent positive change?

Once you have let go of the chaos of trauma, how will you know that you are once again connected to your deepest SELF? When building your goals, you will need to find a way to embrace and celebrate this new you. You will have changed and you will have let go of many traumas—lifted many anchors. How will you celebrate the changes and how will you incorporate them into a brand-new outlook?

But what if you don't change the story? What will it cost you to remain this way?

As humans, we plod along. We are constantly reminded of where we fit in the pecking

Nothing happens when you do nothing; everything stays the same except the problem gets worse.

order of life. We are exhausted from healing and energy work and that is just how it is. We hide from the world because the energies of others drain us and that is just how it is. We want to quit working in our passion but we know that we can't because others need us. We can't take the time to put ourselves first and foremost because to do so would be selfish and would be seen as an insult to those we are here to serve.

What happens if you decide right now that you are going to do nothing?

Nothing happens when you do nothing. Everything stays the same except the problem gets worse. You become more exhausted and further burned out. You draw further into yourself until your circle of close family and friends is non-existent. Your social life becomes a thing of the past. Eventually, you will quit working as a healer and energy worker because your energy will no longer attract people to you. You will suffer physically, emotionally, mentally, and spiritually.

Understanding the root of the problem allows you to gain some perspective. Deciding to take the problem in hand and deal with it now is far less painful than the cost of doing nothing. To do nothing will eventually cost you everything.

If you have decided that you are worth more, that the benefits of solving this problem far outweigh the cost of keeping it, turn the page and let's talk about the work.

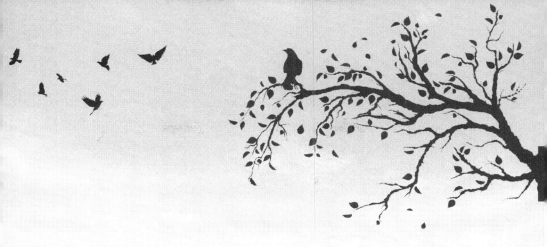

Raising
The Anchor

Have you ever noticed that it is so much easier to do healing work on others and to support them as they work on themselves than it is to turn inward? The idea of putting ourselves and our needs first

The idea of putting ourselves and our needs first and foremost in our lives is a foreign concept to many people, especially healers.

and foremost in our lives is a foreign concept to many people, especially healers. And yet, it is the key to this chapter and this entire model.

You have already delved into what you thought the problem was and explored how it is affecting not only your work as a healer and energy worker, but every single area of your life. You have seen the suffering and pain that has been caused in your life and you can imagine what it will cost you to continue this way. Maybe you are now thinking about yourself and have even set goals that you would like to achieve around letting this suffering go and learning a new way to be. Are you curious about who you will be on the other side of trauma? What are the possibilities and opportunities that will open up for you as you transition from working in your passion to living it and finding the balance with the rest of your life?

The soul has brought along traumas from other lifetimes to live out what was left unresolved.

This next step, I simply call *The Work*. It seems daunting, but don't fret. I won't abandon you down there with the anchor. In fact, this chapter is all about weighing (or raising) the anchor and moving with the flow of life once more. This chapter explains how to work this problem out of your life along with the negative consequences that are currently attached to it. Think of this chapter as the springboard to freedom; the freedom to choose a new way, a new idea, a new you.

In the last chapter, I began the framework for a new perspective—a new light on an old problem. New perspectives often take us out of our comfort zone.

In terms of the core system, the soul is here to live out what it was pre-determined in spirit to be before this life began; the human body is here to accommodate that experience through living. As mentioned in a previous chapter, many people are born into this world with a SELF that is not intact. The soul has brought along traumas from other lifetimes to live out what was left unresolved. The impact of unresolved trauma is then lived out in a mess of humanness and emotion.

When a child is born into the world with a soul that has unresolved traumas from past lives, the core system of the child is already compromised. Some people go through their entire life not realizing that some of their problems are not even of this life. The majority of people never realize that they have the opportunity to release those problems and that they are the leading expert when it comes to doing just that.

There are many things that are within us that we were never taught about or that we were programmed or conditioned to pay no attention to. We have been robbed of an immense opportunity to self-heal, simply by the very nature of our programming. We have been told that what can't be seen or tangibly understood is not relevant—that some forms of healing and energy work are not real. People often refer to the work of self-healing as *Woo Woo* because it is not completely understood. I prefer to call it my passion or my work.

In the work that I do, I work in close conjunction with the soul and with *age* and *past life regression*. For those of you who are unfamiliar with these terms, they simply mean mentally and emotionally going back in time. In order to release a trauma that has affected you deeply and in many areas of your life, you first must understand from where the trauma stems. Going back in time, working with a professional hypnotherapist who will guide you to the exact moment of trauma, will allow insights you couldn't imagine. (Some of my clients are sure that they know what the cause of their trauma is and once they have been guided back to the root, they find it was something completely different.) The point is this—whatever the root of the trauma, you can be guided there. Once you have done the healing work described above, the trauma can be turned around until it is a memory that no longer affects you negatively. Being able to hold onto your memories without emotional triggers, negative cords, or anchors is a truly freeing feeling.

I start with guiding the client back to the time just before they were born, to dismantle and rebuild the foundation that they were born with. This is considered rebuilding the foundation of life from a place of absolute balance and self-love. The client chooses to plant the seed of self-love that will be the foundation that they will work from throughout our work together.

> *A trigger takes us all the way back to the way we felt, reacted to and coped with the initial event.*

This process includes things like nourishing the *inner child*—which is simply catering to that part of us that never grows up. The inner child intermixes with trauma and splinters like shards of broken glass, leaving pieces of itself at the root of every trauma. Because the inner child is not human, it can and does do this. Nourishing the inner child is simply catering to it by showering it with love and healing the wounds it has suffered as a result of the traumas it has endured. A happy inner child lends itself to a balanced overall SELF.

A *trigger* is an event that sinks an anchor further into the sand. Triggers are created when an initial trauma occurs. Following that event, whenever similar circumstances arise, these triggers are reinforced. Triggers take us all the way back to the way we felt, reacted to and coped with the initial event. They compound feelings and emotions so that actions and reactions worsen over time. Because everything is energy and all energy is connected, every single experience in our lives is connected by energetic cords. How we do one thing is how we do all things and what a tangled web has been woven due to unresolved trauma. Can you see more clearly how every part of your life has been impacted by what you thought had only been one part?

> The energetic cords that make up the matrix of our stories connect everything to every other thing in our lives.

The *energetic cords* that make up the matrix of our stories connect everything to every other thing in our lives. In order to release trauma, all of the cords attached to that trauma from all of the experiences in our lives need to be addressed. Some require repair, others healing, and some require cutting. This allows the trauma to be released in all of the ways that is has affected us.

A large part of the work that needs to take place is healing the inner child, releasing triggers, and cutting cords. These all require forgiveness—forgiveness of self and forgiveness of others. Once these issues have been raised and released with forgiveness from a strong foundation of self-love, they are gone for good. Imagine a whole group of joined files on a computer getting flushed as the system is reset. The same happens in this situation. The negative is released and a positive reframe is introduced, allowing for a different story to take hold; one that is in alignment with your goals and your expected outcomes for balance and harmony.

All of the aforementioned release work in this process of the work is accomplished through age and past life regression.

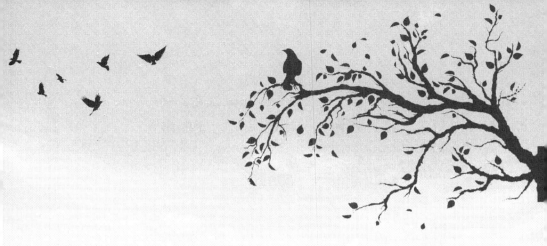

The Soul

Addressing the soul is the final piece of this deconstruction and rebuilding process. Holistically, we can do the release work mentioned above in all areas of body, mind, soul.

> *Soul retrieval is the act of bringing the soul back to a whole once again.*

The soul is a special place. Here we are working with a pure energy. Working with the soul is about ensuring optimal connection and communication with the core system and spirit. The soul, when in balance in the core, lends to a more carefree and balanced SELF.

Sometimes when the core system is out of balance, the soul does a little splintering of its own. This is referred to as soul loss or fragmentation. *Soul retrieval* is that act of bringing the soul back to a whole once again. Often, this step alone brings about the balance that is required in the core system.

Soul retrieval is referred to as soul hunting in Shamanic practice and refers to bringing back parts of the soul that were lost. In many cultures worldwide, there is a belief that sickness and suffering happen because parts of the soul have gone

A soul pod is a group of deeply interconnected souls who travel together as a group through multiple lifetimes.

missing. Soul retrieval is of the utmost importance in maintaining homeostasis within the core and out into the rest of the body.

Souls are multi-dimensional sources of energy. Before they choose to incarnate into a human host, souls choose what traumas are to be lived out in the hope that they will be dealt with in the lifetime they have chosen.

Have you ever met an individual or a group of people for the first time and you just knew that these people were your people—on the same vibe as you? Some refer to this as their *tribe*. Perhaps you have even collaborated with your *people* on projects that have brought about great change, understanding, or healing. These people are likely part of your soul pod. A *soul pod* is a group of souls who travel together as a group through multiple lifetimes and are deeply interconnected. Soul pods work together for a common purpose. Ignoring the urge you have to join your soul pod will cause trauma in the form of loneliness and isolation.

A soul contract is an agreement made with another soul prior to birth.

Do you have a soul mate? Do you long for that one person who will complete you in this lifetime? If you feel or have ever felt this way, it is likely that you have a soul contract with another soul. A *soul contract* is an agreement made with another soul prior to birth. The contract allows for a very deep connection between two souls and will also likely bring about deep changes as well. To ignore the soul contract is to cause trauma in your life in the form of loneliness, a constant feeling of missing a piece of yourself, and profound disconnection.

Many of my clients have come to me with questions about their soul mate. Some feel they know who that individual is in this lifetime and others have been searching without any success. It has been my experience that many of my clients do have soul mates and have encountered these souls in past life regressions. These individuals have reincarnated over lifetimes to cross each other's path on the life journey. Others have a soul mate in which the relationship (or relationships) from past lives has not necessarily been positive. There is a reincarnation, however, the relationships tend to be more volatile and there is more opportunity for separation of the soul mates.

There is a certain way that you have lived this life of yours until now, certain patterns, habits, beliefs, fears and phobias. When we are small children, we learn from the world around us how to live and how to survive as humans. But as we grow older, we may branch out on our own, challenging the status quo and changing our lives to suit what has been innately programmed in. Do you realize that even this way in which we live comes from the soul?

> *Soul vows are written prior to birth and transferred from the soul to the human host at birth to serve as a blueprint of how to walk this earth.*

Soul vows are written prior to birth and transferred from the soul to the human host at birth to serve as a blueprint of how to walk this earth daily. This blueprint involves how to live with authenticity and integrity, how to show up in relationships, and how to partner with universal energy to create a whole life.

These vows are not said as we understand the word vows to mean. Rather soul vows *are* you. They become you and you become them—and as you do, you gather the living presence of universal energy through you and as you.

Aligning the soul and its many aspects is key to releasing the cause of your problems. The soul is where we receive all direction for the human existence we are living. In order for this direction to be crystal clear, balance, connection and communication must remain sharp.

Now that we have gone through what is involved with releasing trauma, I don't want you to lose heart or hope. In later chapters, I will explain just how simple and easy this process can and will be for you.

There is a great deal to process with releasing trauma. You have spent years building that trauma and your resulting problem, so how could you possibly think that it could be as simple as willing it to go away? I understand that thought process well because I was there once too. Then I found an easier, deeper and more permanent way to release all the traumas and their concurrent issues and to write a brand-new story that is filled with my own goals and positive outcomes.

In the next chapter, we will discuss how once you have released what you don't want—you can get to the business of building what you want instead.

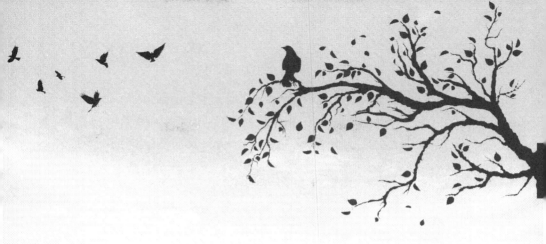

Restoring Balance

Once an anchor has been lifted, you are no longer stuck to the floor in that old story. The last chapter was about letting go and laying a new foundation. The hard work is now done. This chapter is

The page is blank … and you are holding the pen. Welcome to the new you, the new story of your life

about balancing your inside world and living it in the outer world. Now you can create the conditions for success, and live the life you have always wanted.

The page is blank… and you are holding the pen. Welcome to the new you, the new story of your life.

Once we have released trauma and negativity, we can start rebuilding from a solid foundation of self-love. This requires getting back to the basics of life and ensuring that our needs are being met. According to Anthony Robbins (entrepreneur, best-selling author, philanthropist, life and business strategist) there are six basic life necessities. For the purposes of achieving balance, it is important to understand how these areas intersect.

The six basic needs and their characteristics are:

- Certainty: safety, security, stability, comfort, control
- Variety: challenge, excitement, adventure, change, surprise
- Significance: meaning, importance, worthiness
- Connection to others: approval of and attachment to others
- Growth: emotional, intellectual, spiritual development
- Contribution: serving, protecting, caring

The first four (certainty, variety, significance, connection to others) are the needs of the personality and so this means that they deal with our humanness. The last two needs (growth and contribution) are the needs of the soul.

When the six basic needs are working harmoniously with each other, there is a balance at the deepest level of SELF. All of the characteristics of these basic needs are lived out through human experience. For instance, an example of imbalance would be the individual who is constantly seeking significance in the larger world and then having trouble finding connections and deeper relationships with others.

Another example of imbalance would be the healer who is finding that their offerings are being passed over for new modalities, but refuses to keep up with new practices and techniques—thereby stagnating their own growth and success.

One example I like to reference when I have clients whose work is all consuming: it is often our need to feel like we are making a significant difference and that we are contributing to our organization at the expense of our own personal lives. But, if suddenly that work is taken away, as a result of either job loss or retirement, there is often a huge sense of imbalance. Our security and significance are no longer there. If the void comes through job loss, previous workplace contribution seems to be unappreciated and it is often difficult to focus on the other areas of life with the same vigor.

In my practice, I ask the hypnotized client's higher mind to scale the six basic needs from one to ten, one being completely out of balance and ten being balanced and working harmoniously. If any or all of the needs are not at a ten, then it is a simple matter of asking the client's higher mind to bring them to ten and into balance. Once the client has released the traumas, their mind very quickly latches onto new ideas that are of benefit moving forward. In other words, the mind wants more of what feels good. My clients have experienced immediate effects from this shift.

When in balance, the basic needs allow the client to be supported outwardly as they feel what it is like to stand in their own personal power and to feel that energy as it corrects and self-adjusts within them.

In chapter five, we discussed the nine key traits of the SELF:

- Self-Love: regard for one's own happiness
- Self-Confidence: trust in one's own abilities, qualities, judgements
- Self-Esteem: confidence in one's own worth and ability (also referred to as Self-Respect)
- Self-Worth: one's perceived value or worth as a person

- Self-Image: perception of one's abilities, appearance, personality
- Self-Acceptance: perception of one's strengths and weaknesses
- Self-Awareness: conscious knowledge of one's character and feelings
- Self-Actualization: the fulfillment of one's talents, gifts and potentials (considered to be what drives us from within)
- Self-Care: care and attention paid to one's body, mind and spirit

Contrary to popular belief, the SELF and its traits are not developed as we move through life. Rather they are brought into this life and melded between the soul and the human. This means that the soul delivers the SELF and its traits to us prior to birth. All of our traits stem from the deepest part of us— the SELF—and work in conjunction the core system.

When the SELF is not in balance or when even the smallest tear in the web of the SELF occurs, there has been a trauma of some kind. All trauma comes from inside and all trauma stems from an imbalance or disconnection from the deepest SELF.

In my practice, I use a scale from one to ten (one being low and ten being high) to find out with my client just where the imbalance is occurring. Simply asking that each and every area of the SELF be brought to ten and into full balance by the client's higher mind nets immediate positive results—as this is where true personal power lies and along with it, the power of your voice.

Once the basic needs are at ten and the traits of the SELF are at ten, the client experiences an immediate shift. The body, mind and soul adjust to release anything and everything that is

The higher mind has done the work to create the conditions for nothing less than success.

no longer serving the needs of the client. All traumas and any remnants that are left after doing the work are released. The client is elevated to a place of complete personal power once again. I have witnessed an immediate physical difference in posture and energy when this system is brought into balance.

By connecting this new energy from the soul to the body, new synergy and harmony are created, causing immediate higher connection and communication between the spirit and the core. The higher mind has done the work to create the conditions for nothing less than success.

Earlier, I wrote: how we do one thing is how we do all things. When we make a change in one area of our lives, we make changes in all. Once all negative has been released, healing can be invited into all levels of the *actual body*—including the physical, emotional, mental,and spiritual bodies of the human. This healing will align with the balance that has been achieved at the deepest level of SELF and will shift, adjust and optimize for the benefit of continual and effective connection and communication between the soul and the human body. This is the area where clients notice the majority of shifts as the actual body aligns with the soul. We will discuss these shifts further in the next chapter.

The last piece of balance to achieve is in the unseen. The unseen—or spirit—is personally my favorite work to do. The unseen work involves working with spiritual energy, connecting with the core system, and bringing everything into alignment:

The *chakra system* (a complex network of energy channels or spiritual nervous system) is assessed to ensure that it is functioning optimally as are the meridians (energy networks of the body; channels through which energy flows) of the body.

The *aura* (an egg-shaped, electromagnetic, coloured energy field that encompasses the body) is cleansed, reset, and repaired.

There are *morphic fields* (natural systems within the body with inherent memory which become more powerful through repetition). Morphic fields will either need to be attached to or detached from in your best interest. This involves raising your own frequencies and vibrations to allow for that continuous inner balance.

Familial methylation (the stuff that we inherit from the gene pool of our family members) will also be addressed, releasing anything and everything that is no longer necessary. At the same time, your cultural, ancestral, genetic, and cellular memories will be assessed and optimized for your benefit and highest outcome.

Once all of these areas have been addressed and are working for the client's best interest, "the work" has been completed, and remaining remnants of your "don't wants" have been removed, there are two tasks left.

Task One: Now that you have seen the body of work that is involved with tearing down and then rebuilding, would you be willing to take the risk of falling back into old habits? My guess is that you are shaking your head with a hard NO. Why would anyone want to slip back into the old habit of feeling exhausted and burned out?

Task one is a question for your higher mind to answer: *"Can I now release the habit of having these issues altogether? Yes or No?"*

The *habit of having an issue* simply means the pattern or habit that we had previously been living in. As humans, we all have habits that we live in everyday and they go largely unnoticed—even if they are detrimental—until we address trauma and release it. This release then causes shifting in our body, mind and soul and some old habits are no longer necessary.

If the answer is yes, then the habit of having this problem is released. If the answer is no, then either more work may be required or another problem may have surfaced. If another problem has surfaced, the higher mind will go back and assess all of the work that has been done—ensuring that everything is released before then also releasing the habit of having this issue.

Task Two: Think back to chapter one and the person that you were then. Did you like that person? Did you like how you felt and the shape that your life was taking? If you are here now, I am willing to bet that the person in chapter one is not the person that you wish to remain. That person has a set of *identities* that do not align with your highest potential, highest good or benefit, and certainly not with the goals and outcomes that you have set for yourself.

Once you have chosen to release the habit of having these issues once and for all, follow through with task two.

Task two is a question for your higher mind to answer: *"Can I now release the identities created by having these issues? Yes or No?"*

If the answer is yes, then the identities created by having this problem are released. If the answer is no, then either more work may be required or another problem may have surfaced. If another problem has surface, the higher mind will go back and assess all of the work that has been done—ensuring that everything is released before then also releasing the identities created by having this issue.

These two questions can seem monumental as you read them. After all, we are talking about years and years and even lifetimes of trauma and the resulting list of problems and issues. However, at this point in the process, you will have done a huge body of work, both in releasing the old and unwanted and building a new foundation that holds no place for any of the old and unwanted. All of this work has been done by you and for you; I was just the guide and support—it is you who picked up the pen.

These two questions are actually very simple and take very little thought at all. As humans, we are creatures of pleasure and pleasure comes from what feels the best to us, and we usually choose what feels best to us at the time. When faced with living in a continuous state of upheaval and trauma as compared to a clean slate that allows for balance and positive growth toward your own personal goals, what feels more pleasurable to you?

Once you have done the work, balance is restored. Congratulations! You are now holding the pen to write the new story of your life.

So how will you know that you are on the right track? What are the signs that something has actually taken place, even though you may not see it right away? How will you recognize that healing has occurred or is in the process of occurring?

How will you gauge whether or not you have achieved or are working in the direction of your desired outcomes?

How will you maintain this new you?

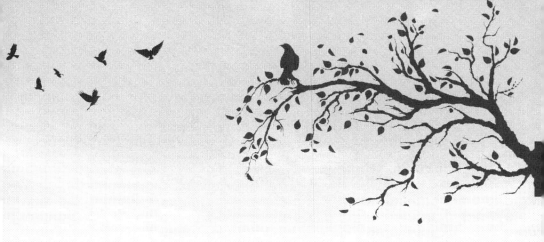

Recognizing Reconnection

A satisfied life is better than a successful life. Our success is measured by others but our satisfaction is measured within. There is a level of peace and gratitude that

> *A satisfied life is better than a successful life; our success is measured by others, but our satisfaction is measured within.*

settles into our lives when we are satisfied with our progress. Success becomes more about others as we start to share the secrets of our own success. Working in our passion as healers and energy workers is no longer a chore. We allow energies to exchange without overwhelming us and, as a result of this lack of inhibition, we end up serving those who are in need of us in a much higher capacity.

When we are satisfied, all things become easier in all areas of our lives. How we do one thing is how we do all things and when one thing gets better, it all gets better.

You have a calming effect on others as you yourself are working at a higher frequency, and from a new place of clarity, focus, and personal power.

Physically, the body will make the changes necessary to create the conditions for balance within. You may notice aches and pains are gone, symptoms of dis-ease are lessened or have completely vanished, and your body may respond in different and more appropriate ways to outside stimulus. You may even notice improvements in your complexion and your hair. Some notice that they were experiencing the weight loss that they had always wanted. One client of mine walked away from cigarettes completely overnight. Let me just say that there will be changes and they will be exactly what you need.

With this new clarity, you are more focused, attentive and caring for yourself in ways that you never thought to before.

Emotionally, the mind will alter how you act and react in any given situation and you may notice that you are not experiencing the highs and lows of the emotional roller coaster that had previously been your life. When you are working with others, you may realize that you are no longer taking on their emotional roller coaster. In fact, your demeanor has a calming effect on them as you yourself work at a higher frequency, and from a new place of clarity, focus, and personal power.

Mentally, the brain fog will lift. You will feel better and will have clarity of thought. Perhaps you will find that with this new clarity, you are more focused, attentive and caring for yourself in ways that you never thought to before. Heaviness and depressive thoughts are no longer normal as you move forward because you now have focus and control and you know what you want and how that will look. Mentally, you may find that all of the beliefs that you had previously settled for that had been anchoring you are no longer there. The memory of how you had coped in the past comes and goes as only a fleeting memory.

Spiritually, your body's chakra system and meridians will automatically align, your aura will cleanse and repair itself. You will find yourself vibrating at a higher frequency—one that is in alignment with the desired outcomes for balance and harmony that you had hoped for at the beginning of this process. As a spiritual worker, you find yourself with a stronger connection to and increased ability to commune with your sources.

You may find that now you have changed, so has your clientele. Those who seek you out now for healing and energy work are on a different journey. They have goals and they know where they want

You have created a different set of standards and your internal blueprint has changed.

to end up. You may find that those energies that completely drained you in the past no longer present themselves to you. Because your vibration is higher and you have a newer, stronger, and more protected sense of self, the universe may conspire to send you only those who truly need your help and healing.

At first, this shift in both your personal and client relationships may seem somewhat scary and isolating. When you make huge changes in your own life and start to vibrate higher, some people will fall away from you because they are no longer on your wave length. You have created a different

> *There will be those who had moved away from you who will resurface in your life.*

set of standards and your internal blueprint has changed. Many people who are stuck will move away from you because they want change but fear change at the same time. Some people are so stuck that they have the belief that others can and will change and move on but that they are not deserving of the same freedom. Just know that some will stay in your circle and some will go and that it is okay to let that happen.

In the same breath, there will be those who had moved away from you who will resurface in your life. There will be new faces as well. These people recognize your vibration and are at the same level as you. They will support you, comfort you, teach you, learn from you—and they will not drain you because there is nothing to take from you.

People come into our lives for many reasons. One is that they will become your *people*—those you vibe with (also known as your *tribe*). They are aligned with you as you start to write the story of this new life.

There are another group of people in your life and these are the ones you will find that just fall away, some quickly and some over time. These people are the takers, the energy vampires and they are stuck. It is not up to you to carry them. Allow them to go, send them with blessings. One day, they may find the pen that writes their new story as well and they will return. If not, it is okay.

This chapter is about how to recognize that a change has taken place and to gauge whether or not you have reached a level of satisfaction that is working for you. It is about recognizing that you are moving from a fixed (have or don't have) to a growth (able to develop) mindset. Gaining and losing people in your life at this time of shift is all part of the change and it will be seamless.

In thinking about the goals that you set for yourself, where do you expect your desired outcomes to lie?

If you choose the fixed mindset (have or don't have), you are limiting yourself (me or others), and continuing to live the way you always have—continuing with the old story of your life.

> *Reconnection to the deepest SELF allows you to make choices that had previously been shielded from you.*

However, if you choose a growth mindset (able to develop), the sky is the limit, the page is blank, and you are holding the pen. A closed mind sees nothing but the old story. An open mind finds a new pen, and begins to write fresh material.

Reconnection to the deepest SELF allows you to make choices that had previously been shielded from you. It allows you to live the choice that you have made to put yourself first and foremost in your own life and to realize that when you do, your relationships with others improve.

When one is standing in their power and using their voice in an impactful way, it becomes easy to realize goals and to build on them. There are new thoughts and ideas that seemingly come from nowhere and everything is done with strength and courage and love. Others around recognize that power and respond to it by either falling away or rising up to meet it. You are more impactful, getting better outcomes for you and for those you were meant to serve. *Reconnection allows you to fully realize that it is not me or them but rather we are all one.*

Reconnection to SELF breaks all the old patterns. It allows you to toss the old story of your life—as you stand in a new place with a new pen. It shatters the patterns of imbalance, dis-ease and suffering in your life. Old traumas have been moved out along with the negative attachments to them, leaving room for personal, positive growth.

Reconnection to SELF works to activate your authentic self, releasing anything and everything that is not—and was never—you to begin with.

I know first-hand of this profound *Reconnection to SELF* as I have gone through this process myself. One day, my Mum told me a story about how when I was a little girl there were two of me living in one body. One was the person that was my true self and the other was the angry, fearful, and envious person who was not truly me. Mum told me that for many years she worried about me because the untrue me was really strong and was allowed to live my life for me. I pushed away friends, family and many opportunities because I was angry, fearful, and envious of others' lives. In an effort to have the life I saw others living, I constantly changed my mind and how I presented myself to the outside world. She told me that I couldn't even see the damage I was doing and the toll it was taking—not only on me, but also on others. Eventually, many of my friends and family left my life.

After too many years of living a life of self-loathing and loneliness, I am happy to say that today the *untrue* me is no longer in charge. I have all of the memories of that time in my life, but I have chosen a different and much more honoring path for myself. I did the work of reconnection to my deepest SELF and when I did, my old story was done. The last page was written and the book was closed.

In my new story, and from a solid foundation of self-love, I am true to myself and I am able to stand in my own

> *Reconnection to SELF restructures your core system, creating balance, harmony, and a strong sense of life purpose.*

personal power and use my voice. The story I write now is one of choice and infinite opportunity because I have a balance within myself. I am now my own best friend. The memories from my old story serve only to strengthen, encourage, and inspire me as I continue to move away from what I don't want and toward what I do. I am grateful to that old life now that I am no longer living the story because it has helped to shape the true me.

Reconnection to SELF changes your perception—how you live in your world. Your senses are reprogrammed so that you approach the way you live and interact in the world in healthy, more positive ways. *Reconnection to SELF* restructures your core system, creating balance, harmony, and a strong sense of life purpose. With all of these shifts inside the body, perceptions of others and the outside world have to change as well.

Reconnection to SELF makes shifts and changes throughout the body, mind and soul—even restructuring our cells and DNA to allow for support and personification of our authentic self in the outside world.

> *The results of deeper healing are often noticed by those around you before you realize them for yourself.*

There is healing available to you on all levels of body, mind and soul—both superficially and at a deeper level. Superficial healing refers to those things you may notice right away. Perhaps you feel lighter, perhaps you are not as tired, or not as anxious as you used to be. Superficial healing is instantaneous and almost unnoticeable unless you are paying attention. Deeper healing is much more pronounced and yet it may be just as unnoticeable. The results of deeper healing are often noticed by those around you before you realize them for yourself.

Some of the signs you are healing at a deep level that others may notice first are that you:

- Are more observant and less judgmental
- Are more responsive and less reactionary
- Are more self-loving and less self-sabotaging
- Have more boundaries with less resentment
- Have more inner peace with less outer chaos
- Have more clarity and less confusion
- Are more just being and less doing
- Have more faith and less fear.

Don't be surprised if these signs are noticed by others who know you best before you notice them for yourself. All of these signs mean that you are putting yourself first and foremost in your life. By standing in your power, you are choosing to live a different way. People will notice a change in you even if you don't recognize it yourself. When they do and bring it to your attention, all you need to do is reflect on how it feels to act in a different way and then enjoy it.

So, what now? Now that you have solved this problem, how do you maintain this level of "what you want instead"? In the next chapter, we will discuss maintaining this level of feel good.

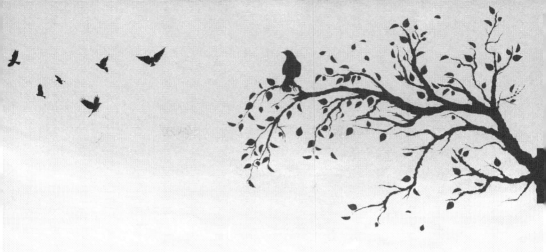

Next Steps

By now you have probably realized that maintaining the new story of your life requires work and finesse. The story is going to be continuous just as your old story was and so it is important to keep writing forward. The soul is a pure thing and the SELF, when balanced, works in absolute harmony with the soul and the rest of the core system. The challenge in moving forward is our humanness and our SELF that lies in our humanness.

Have you ever heard of the onion effect? That is when you have solved the bigger problem and are moving forward in new and rewarding ways—but now other things that are wanting your attention have room to come to the surface. Once that layer has been completely peeled away, there is another layer. This is not a bad thing; this is the next step in your new story. When we go through our lives living in trauma, exhaustion, brain fog and burnout, we often focus on the biggest problem at the time. Once that problem has been resolved, life runs smoothly for a while—until another issue makes itself known. Often these other issues are small and sometimes they are fragments of the larger problem that need sorting out. Whatever the new issue, and regardless of its size, it needs attention and work—the very same work you have just done with a larger issue. It is up to you to choose. Will you allow this new issue to fester and grow or will you choose to do maintenance work on this new story that you have started for yourself? Remember, this is all about choice—yours. You are the one holding the pen.

Our traumas are layers of an onion. Once one layer has been completely peeled away, there is another trauma to be dealt with waiting underneath. Now, this isn't something that will go on forever. Just as onions run out of layers, eventually you will run out of issues coming up as well. It is important to acknowledge and recognize that there may be several layers to work through before you have completely achieved your desired outcome of total balance and harmony.

It is one thing to achieve balance and harmony in our inner world and quite another to live in that balance in the outer world.

The human part of us must live this messy and unpredictable thing we call life. It is one thing to achieve balance and harmony in our inner world and quite another to live in that balance in the outer world. People and situations get in the way of our perfection and sometimes serve to test our resolve. According to neuroscientist and philosopher Dr. Deepak Chopra, it is estimated that we have between sixty and eighty thousand thoughts going through our minds on a daily basis. So how do we keep things moving forward in the right direction?

One word—Hypnosis.

We all live in the same world; we all face the realities of being human on a daily basis. However, as opposed to many who live in the world of constructs and concretes, as a hypnotherapist, I live in a world filled with expansion and opportunity.

In the world of hypnosis, I work with the mind, and in particular, the higher mind—that part of us that connects to spiritual energy. This level of the subconscious mind is the most amazing part of ourselves. I work with the blank page that each client brings to me and through the practice of hypnosis, together we create a personal masterpiece by releasing the negative and enhancing the positive. Basically, client-driven change.

I consider hypnosis as simply the language of the mind that serves as a gateway for us to connect to the best and ultimate parts of ourselves.

> *Hypnosis is a choice.*

Hypnosis is a choice. Every individual chooses whether or not to allow themselves to go into trance. Therefore, hypnosis is not sleep, but rather an altered level of consciousness. It is not forgetting; as you are not asleep. In the process of hypnotherapy, you will hear and remember everything that is of importance during the session. It is not loss of control; rather, it is taking full and complete control of your own mind to explore and

> *It is your choice to allow your highest mind to guide you, support you, teach you, and allow you to choose what you accept and what you don't.*

unearth the answers you are seeking to solve your problem in the best way for you.

In my practice working with clients who have chosen to utilize my *Reconnection to SELF* model, I serve as a hypnotic tour guide. I allow you the space to choose to change your life, your circumstances, your habits, patterns and beliefs for the better. It is *your* choice to allow that highest mind of yours to guide you, support you, teach you and allow you to choose what you accept and what you don't. Unlike stage hypnosis where the hypnotist is setting up suggestion in the minds of the participants, my practice in hypnotherapy is holistic and client-centered. This means that the client's higher mind serves as the suggestor, allowing the client to choose to accept or decline their own solutions.

Hypnosis has been proven to be 93% successful after just six sessions. (American Health Magazine).

Our lives are made up of the choices we make and the more we understand about the connection with our highest mind and get into complete trust with it, the better the choices are that we make for permanent positive change. Hypnosis is *You-to-You* therapy—and who knows you better than you? You're the expert.

According to American Health Magazine (February 2007), *Hypnosis has been proven to be 93% effective after just six sessions, in comparison with a 38% success rate after six hundred sessions of psychoanalysis, and a 72% success rate after twenty-two sessions of behavior therapy.* The reason for this is simple—unlike other therapies that deal with clients who are trying to figure out the problem in the conscious mind and relying on willpower for change, hypnosis gets immediately into the subconscious and higher mind and deals with the problem at its root. The conscious mind is the weakest of all levels of the mind and lives in the everyday; it is where willpower and ego live.

The subconscious or higher mind is the all-knowing part of the mind that has the answers we are looking for. Changes made in the higher mind are systemic throughout all levels of body, mind and soul which cause an immediate and sustained effect.

Unlike other therapies that deal with clients who are trying to figure out the problem in the conscious mind and relying on willpower for change, hypnosis gets immediately into the subconscious and deals with the problem at its root.

One comfort for my clients when working with some of these powder keg issues is that I never have to know what's causing the issue or any of the details that the client may not want to share or talk about. The secrets, insecurities and intimate details of their traumas are safe within themselves. They don't have to tell me anything at all if that is what they choose. The client is in control. I don't need to know, and they don't need to relive any of their trauma with me in order to release it completely.

The client knows their own mind and that is what causes the choice for change within—I am just the hypnotic tour guide. It is the client who creates the changes within themselves. It's all about choice—theirs.

It is the client who creates the changes within themselves.

Healing really is an inside job. When large and deep traumas are released, there is healing that needs to take place. Hypnosis allows for unprecedented access to your highest mind where the release of traumas and attached issues are supported systemically with physical, emotional, mental and spiritual healing, as well as soul work.

I did the work for my own healing and growth. I faced the reality that there were areas of my life that I needed to heal. I am grateful every day that I was given the opportunity of my own reconnection to SELF at the deepest level. I am, as all humans are, a continuous work in progress. The difference now is that I am buffing and shining around the edges because the bigger traumas are long gone.

It has been my honor to share my story and this model with you in the hope that you may recognize yourself in it and choose to make a difference in your life as well—to start fresh with a new and improved story of your life.

Are you ready to pick up the pen?

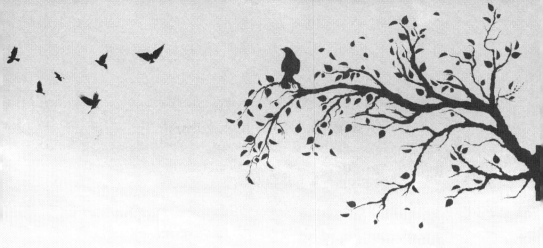

It's About Choice—Not Willpower

We all live in a world filled with choices. Choice—not control—is the only truth that we actually have as humans living in this world. Choice comes with ownership because when we make choices, the results are ours. The problem comes when we make a choice that doesn't align with our truth. When the consequence of that choice goes awry, we then look for someone or something to blame. If we are not careful, this pattern of blaming others will take on a life of its own and soon a trauma starts to form. Once a trauma has formed, it isn't long before it starts to affect everything in our lives, everywhere in our lives. Traumas are the result of a lack of responsibility for the choices we make.

> *Choice—not control—is the only truth that we actually have as humans living in this world.*

As I have mentioned previously, just because we are responsible for the choices we make that lead to a building of trauma, that does not in any way mean that we are responsible for the actions of outside influence that cause us trauma. What we are responsible for is how we choose to deal with our own feelings, emotions, actions and reactions following the initial event that caused the trauma in the first place.

We are responsible for is how we choose to deal with our own feelings, emotions, actions and reactions following the initial event that caused the trauma in the first place.

After forty plus years of writing the wrong story of my life, I realized that I needed to close that book for my own life to change drastically and positively. Once I really got down to thinking about it and asking my own ego to step aside, it took very little time for change to begin and results to be noted. It was work that I did to give myself an opportunity to write a different story.

I gave up on willpower because I realized that it had never worked for me. If I wanted to solve my own problem, I needed to go deeper and feel connected once again. Once I did that, everything changed. My life and everything in it transformed. I thought differently and more powerfully. My emotions were more controlled and I found myself reacting less or not at all to previous negative triggers around me—the stimuli just weren't a focus any longer. I was acting more in tune with my goals—which allowed my energy to naturally vibrate at a higher frequency. I lost people along the way; but those I gained gave me space and support to continue on a positive and powerful track that created expansion and opportunity in my life. I was, and continue to be, extremely grateful for that shift.

I changed my perspective from one of focusing on what I didn't want (which was only serving to bring me more of the same) to one of what I wanted (which allowed for the old ideas, feelings and situations to fall away). Doors that had been previously closed suddenly opened and with them came people, situations, and opportunities that were in alignment with the brand-new story I was writing for myself.

> *Suffering is a choice.*

Suffering is a choice. Believing that feeling the way you do now—exhausted, burned out and ready to quit—is a choice. Stopping yourself from dreaming big and seizing new opportunities is a choice. Healing all of it is a choice. And the choice is yours.

> *When you have truly healed, you will naturally attract those who are ready to do the same and your work will take on an enriched meaning because of it.*

Imagine the changes in your life and work that you could create with a better connection to yourself. Imagine the opportunities that you could create for the people you work with as a result of working from a place of power. The energy created from a positive place is exponentially stronger than the place you are operating from now and so will the results be for the people you work with. When you have truly healed, you will naturally attract those who are ready to do the same and your work will take on an enriched meaning because of it.

Alternatively, choosing to remain the way you are now will burn you out completely and eventually you will have no choice but to quit working in your passion—to continue would take the ultimate toll on you personally and physically. When we choose not to take care of ourselves and to ignore all of the signs that we are living in trauma, our bodies and our minds eventually take over and go into limp mode and then shut down.

But there is another way.

Hypnosis allows us to bypass our own conscious mind (willpower and ego) to get deep within ourselves where all of the answers are waiting to be accessed.

Consciously using willpower allows trauma to grow. We spend an immense amount of time focusing on the problem because willpower requires focus. Eventually, that focus places blinders on us, preventing us from looking for other strategies and the problem consumes us.

Hypnosis allows us to bypass our own conscious mind (willpower and ego) to really get deep within ourselves where all of the answers are waiting to be accessed. Hypnosis allows for the blinders to fall away to expand and illuminate the problem, so that we are able to see how the problem has affected us in all areas of our life. The process of hypnosis allows us to see the real disconnect from our deepest SELF that has occurred as a result.

Reconnection to SELF re-establishes the balance of powerful person and impactful voice.

Many people choose to continue to believe that they will solve their problem on their own by focusing their attention or trying harder; however, they are continuously being shown proof in their own lives that it just isn't working. Things just continue to build and build.

Reconnection to SELF re-establishes the balance of powerful person and impactful voice within you, giving you the choice to live and work in complete harmony.

Reconnection to SELF will change your life and allow you to know yourself in such a profound way that you will wonder why you struggled until now. Growth and opportunity will start to show up in your life in unimaginable ways. Your imagination will have a chance to run wild and you will reap the rewards of *Reconnection to SELF*—the emergence of your authentic self—free of anchors.

It's a simple process. Realize the problem, expand on the issues with a professional and ask for their help. The rest is all about the choices that you make for

> *Our lives are all about the choices we make.*

better outcomes in your own life and for the lives of those you touch from here onward.

Our lives are all about the choices we make. Our spiritual gifts or passions are part of those choices. We can continue to choose others over ourselves and live the consequences of exhaustion and burnout or we can choose another way.

I hope you choose you. When you do, I am here to support you and to bear witness to a brand-new story in the making.

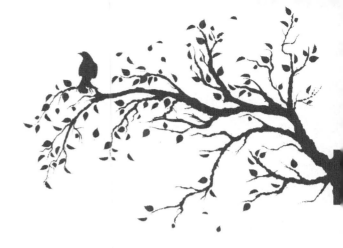

The New Story

Have you ever noticed that when you're finally ready to heal, when you've reached the point where you're ready to create the largest possible shift in your lifetime, that suddenly—rather than seeing threats and obstacles—you start to see everyone and everything around you as a teacher? Do you also notice that often those teachers who are showing up now were people who triggered you in the past?

This book found you for one reason and that is to offer you a solution to your problem. As you read these ideas, you may have realized that the person I am describing throughout is you. This is the story of your life. You are a healer and energy worker and you are tired—beyond tired. You are exhausted emotionally and physically and you have reached the point of burnout. How many times and how badly have you wanted to quit this gift; this passion that lives inside of you and refuses to give you any peace?

When you find yourself walking through hell, your only choice is to keep going because eventually you will choose something different and far less painful.

I know that path. I have been in your shoes and I have tried to quit in the past as well. But something always drew me back and the circus of exhaustion and burnout continued until I found another way. I found a deep solution and created for myself a correction that is positive, powerful, and permanent—allowing me to continue working and living in my passion while feeling fully grounded, protected, and free from any of the old exhaustion and burnout. I now work from and speak from a place of power that comes from within.

My saying goes, "When you find yourself walking through hell, your only choice is to keep going because eventually you will choose something different and far less painful."

That is exactly what happened to me. I found myself by changing my mind and putting myself and my needs first and foremost in my own life and that has made all the difference. I picked up the pen and started writing a new story of my life; one filled with opportunity and balanced from a place of deep personal power.

Once I figured out and solved my own problem, I realized that I had to share this knowledge with others—and so I created the simple model called *Reconnection to SELF*. It allows my clients to see their problem with a fresh perspective and to go deeper within themselves to unearth their own revelations regarding how to solve it.

This new perspective allows for shedding a new light—a lot of new light—on a situation and gives you the opportunity to begin to imagine "what if?". This new perspective also allows you to realize the gravity of the situation that has permeated all areas of your life.

In order to solve a problem, it first must be broken down and dismantled.

And so, the letting go begins. In order to solve a problem, it first must be broken down and dismantled. What isn't necessary any longer is dispersed, leaving room for what comes next—the building phase of things.

We all know what we don't want in our lives and we know the emotions and feelings that come in with what we don't want. In the lifting the anchor phase of the *Reconnection to SELF* model, all of those things are allowed to leave. In their place is space to fill with effective connection and communication

Hypnosis is the fastest, easiest and most permanent way to achieve your goals and desired outcomes.

between the core and the SELF. By optimizing what remains with positive reinforcement around this new connection and communication, you can feel the balance and personal power taking hold and creating a brand-new foundation to stand on. Your voice may even change and become more powerful. These shifts continue to happen and to propel forward motion. At some point, one can feel the closing of the old story and the start of the new story.

Following transition from "what I don't want" to "what I want instead" are signs and cues that you are healing. Most of them will be more obvious to others before they are noticed by you and that is okay. It simply means that you are naturally changing and gravitating to "what you want instead" and it is further verification that your original SELF is once again emerging. All you have to do is to embrace the new you.

Hypnosis is the fastest, easiest and most permanent way to achieve your goals and desired outcomes. Hypnosis allows for a bypass of the conscious mind and willpower. It allows for deep shifts throughout the entire system—soul, body, mind and spirit—in such a way that you will literally say to yourself and others, "I will never be the same again," with a smile on your face and forward momentum in mind.

You will never find the deep healing you are seeking on the outside of yourself.

Healing is an inside job. You will never find the deep healing you are seeking on the outside of yourself. Locked inside your subconscious mind are all of the answers and healing abilities that you will ever need to truly live your passion in the most honoring way possible.

We all live life by choice. We can choose to do what we've always done, expecting a different outcome. We can choose to live with a narrowed view of our lives and our problems which will never lead to growth. Or we can choose to take a chance, to make a choice that will allow the changes we are looking for to come to us in the most seamless way possible.

We are all a work in progress.

We are all a work in progress. For those of us blessed with the gift of healing and service to others, it is imperative that we take better care of ourselves—even better than we do our clients. There is a balance needing to be struck. The choice is ours to write that into our new story.

As we end our time together, my desire for you is that this book has given you a new perspective and has lit your own personal light. There is a power that comes with doing the work at the deepest level of SELF. I have endeavored to give you insight that will allow you to choose to go within yourself to find what you have been searching for.

Knowledge is power and when you understand the power of going within to realize and actualize the SELF, you are in full control of the pen that is writing your story. The only things stopping you from creating that inner strength, to truly stand in the power of your own unique individuality and to find your impactful voice, are the constraints that you have placed on your own imagination.

Step out of your own way.

You are the author of your own unique and beautiful story. If the one you are currently

> *Step out of your own way.*

writing isn't working, if you are stuck or blocked—if your old story is done—set down that pen and close that book. Choose to do your own self work and the new story will start to emerge. All you have to do is pick up the pen.

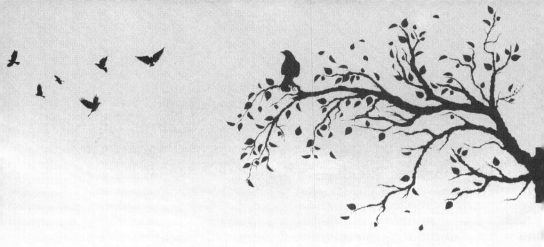

Acknowledgements

First and foremost, I need to send out oceans of thanks to my family. To my partner in crime, Tony, for being the rock that he is and for loving and supporting me in all ways at all times. You are my favorite person ever. Love you Babe! To our children, and many grandchildren, I am so grateful for the joy and inspiration that you have brought to my life and for the belief that you have in me. My life has been shaped and supported by the relationships that I have with all of you and I am richer for it in so many amazing ways.

To my parents and my siblings, thank you for your support and your belief.

Ines Simpson is the creator of *The Simpson Protocol* (Advanced Holistic Hypnosis). She is someone who was originally going to be my teacher but became my family almost instantly. She has been a constant source of support, mentorship and love as our friendship has grown over the past few years. She is constantly reminding me that this life I am living is about me and only *me*. Thank you, my dear friend for your friendship, for your belief, for having the patience and skill to show me how to rescue myself when I didn't know how to do it, and for holding the space while I rewrote my own story. Thank you for always pushing me to go further, to step outside of myself, and to share my gifts with the world. It has been a journey and I am honored to have you walk beside me.

To my *tribe*, I have really no words. Just know that you have all brought so much love, enrichment, joy, laughter, love and support to my life. Special mention to my sister Sian Balogh, and dear friends, Crystal Flood, Gina Strole, Tracy Roy, Linda Boston, Lori Trafford, Sabrina Cote, Joann Gaudreau, Cheryl Tessari, Carole Debreceni, Krista Kirchhofer, Angela Bagu, Kim Baker, Dana Sproat, Paula Swanson, and Patty Meier. You ladies are all earth angels and you have blessed my life in so many ways. You *are* my *tribe* and I love you all!

Acknowledgment and blessings to my angel in heaven, Vickie Kertai. I love you, I miss you, I carry you in my heart.

To all of my friends and colleagues in the HypnoCommunity—please never stop doing what you do. You all inspire me every day! You ROCK! Keep adding your magic to the matrix!

And last but certainly not least, I'd like to mention fellow author and friend, Denise Anderson, who has been on the sidelines encouraging me through this journey. Thank you for all of your support my friend. Your energy is pure dynamite and I love it!

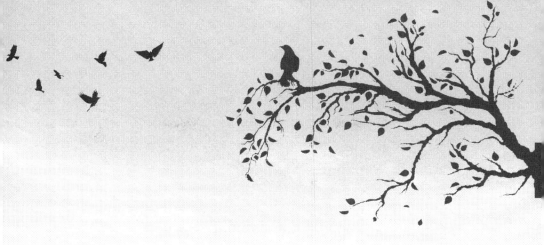

About the
Author

Jacquie Balogh is a Certified Clinical Hypnotherapist, trainer, medium, speaker and author who specializes in Advanced Holistic Hypnosis. Her passion and focus are on moving her clients past willpower and into personal power to rewrite the story of their lives. Jacquie's first book, (The Burned-Out Healer ~ A Path to Trauma 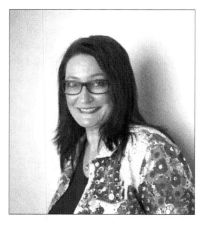 Release & Reconnection to SELF) lays the groundwork for self-healing and self-connection while navigating through the personal burnout of energy healing.

Jacquie's absolute passion is to see people on their own path in life in balance and harmony. In her work, she seeks to empower and support people to stand in their own unique individuality and to encourage them to find the power of their own voice and their own personal path. Jacquie's greatest achievement is to have people see that they are more than enough and that they have everything inside of themselves to change their world and the world around them.

Jacquie's background in licensed practical nursing as well as certifications in Reiki Mastery, Conflict Management, Sacred Gifts, Wellness Coaching, Hypnotherapy and Advanced Hypnotherapy resulting from her own personal healing journey have enriched her life in many aspects. She has a compassionate, open-minded and matter of fact approach with everyone she comes into contact with. She offers simple, easy to incorporate solutions that have given her clients fresh perspectives and a new pen time and again. She believes in keeping things simple while getting straight to the heart of the matter.

Jacquie lives and works in Calgary, Alberta, Canada but knows that there are no borders to stop her from working in her passion for helping and healing others. She has a thriving global online practice. She has also undertaken teaching *The Simpson Protocol Hypnosis*—both live and online—to other hypnotists and enthusiasts alike as Canada's first certified trainer.

Jacquie works with everything and anything and believes that whatever comes her way was meant to be. If you have a problem, you have a solution—and she is always ready and willing to help you get there.

"There are only two times in our lives;
NOW and TOO LATE.

But if it's "NEVER TOO LATE,"
then all we really have is right NOW!"

~ Jacquie Balogh

THANKS FOR READING

It is with love and gratitude that I say thank you for choosing my book (The Burned-Out Healer ~ A Path to Trauma Release & Reconnection to SELF).

By now you have decided whether or not to pick up the pen and to re-write the story of your life. It is my passion and my pleasure to support you in making this monumental decision to fill the blank pages.

I've created a companion session for this book and would love to invite you to email me to book your one-on-one appointment with me. This session further assists with both guiding and supporting you as you make the very best choices for yourself.

I am excited for you...

Get your pen ready!

Email: jacquie@transcendencehypnosis.com